SPINAL CORD INJURY

Concepts and Management Approaches

SPINAL CORD INJURY
Concepts and Management Approaches

Lorraine E. Buchanan, R.N., M.S.N.

Project Coordinator
Regional Spinal Cord Injury Center of Delaware Valley
Thomas Jefferson University
Philadelphia, Pennsylvania

Deborah A. Nawoczenski, M.Ed., P.T.

Assistant Professor
Department of Physical Therapy
Temple University
Philadelphia, Pennsylvania

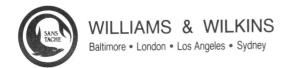

WILLIAMS & WILKINS
Baltimore • London • Los Angeles • Sydney

Editor: John Butler
Associate Editor: Victoria M. Vaughn
Copy Editor: Gail N. Chalew
Design: JoAnne Janowiak
Illustration Planning: Asterisk Group
Production: Anne G. Seitz

Copyright © 1987
Williams & Wilkins
428 East Preston Street
Baltimore, MD 21202, U.S.A.

96900

Printed in the United States of America

Library of Congress Cataloging in Publication Data

Main entry under title.

Spinal cord injury.

Includes index.
1. Spinal cord—Wounds and injuries. 2. Spinal cord—Wounds and injuries—
Patients—Rehabilitation. I. Buchanan, Lorraine E. II. Nawoczenski, Deborah A.
[DNLM: 1. Spinal Cord Injuries—therapy. WL 400 S757] RD594.3.S6687
1987   617′.482044   86-13289
ISBN 0-683-06176-3

Composed and printed at the
Waverly Press, Inc.

87 88 89 90 91
10 9 8 7 6 5 4 3 2 1

Foreword

Hopes for persons with spinal cord injury have improved dramatically over the past 40 years. In the United States, although there was a relatively small group of dedicated professionals interested in spinal cord injury after World War II, the interest did not really become widespread until about 15 years ago. This interest was generated by the combined efforts of health professionals and persons in government, and led to a decision by the Rehabilitation Service Administration to develop and fund comprehensive centers for the care of persons with spinal cord injury. This catalyzed a chain reaction that improved the outlook for these people. A system of care had to encompass all aspects of management, including emergency medical services, acute medical care, rehabilitation, discharge planning, community support, and long-term follow-up. Adjuncts to medical care included psychological, social, and vocational support. Obviously, this effort required the interest and help of many health care professionals. Because spinal cord injury became a recognized problem that needed attention, educational programs and research became popular. The interest and participation by many allied health professionals from various disciplines led to a truly comprehensive team approach to provide the broad spectrum of services needed by persons with spinal cord injury. Team members focused on the whole patient and became quite knowledgeable about many aspects of spinal cord injury care.

This book, which has been written by and for allied health professionals, illustrates the depths of knowledge of many of these team members. It provides an important educational resource that can further stimulate interest, training, and research in the field of spinal cord injury. The unfortunate person with a spinal cord injury requires a well-educated and well-balanced team to meet his needs and to assist him in attaining a reasonable quality of life until a more definitive cure can be found.

Samuel L. Stover, M.D.

Preface

Spinal Cord Injury: Concepts and Management Approaches is intended to serve the allied health professional as a guide to the care of the person with spinal cord injury from the time of injury through lifetime follow-up. It provides a basis for understanding the devastating challenge that traumatic spinal cord injury presents to the injured person, his or her family and significant others, the health care community, and society.

This book is not intended to replace procedure manuals that are available in most institutions serving large numbers of spinal cord injured patients. Indeed, a deliberate attempt has been made to address the issues related to traumatic spinal cord injury and not to utilize a "how to" format. We have also chosen to focus on management approaches without addressing specific role responsibilities of each professional.

It is our hope that concerned allied health professionals will build upon the basic concepts presented here to develop specific management strategies that will be most effective and appropriate within their institutional settings. Often there are several different methods and strategies that can be utilized to achieve the same goal. It is most important to recognize the goal and the potential obstacles that may prevent the injured person from achieving it. For that reason, we have attempted to suggest strategies for consideration and, wherever possible, not to infer that there is only one correct approach.

We have been fortunate to involve a group of superb clinicians as contributing authors. Each one was chosen for his or her experience and proven expertise in spinal cord injury rehabilitation and related fields. We thank each of them for their invaluable contributions.

Lorraine E. Buchanan, R.N., M.S.N.
Deborah A. Nawoczenski, M.Ed., P.T.

Acknowledgments

We are fortunate that very talented and dedicated professionals have assisted us with the preparation of this manuscript. We wish to express special thanks to our contributing authors for sharing their expertise in the team concept of spinal cord injury management.

We are grateful to Dr. Samuel Stover for giving his valuable time to provide the forward to this text. Thanks also to Dr. Jerome Cotler, professor of orthopedics and co-associate director of acute care of the Regional Spinal Cord Injury Center of Delaware Valley, for his input in the chapters on acute management. Appreciation is also extended to our typist, Gisele Hamilton; our photographer, Lawrence Albee; our illustrator, Joyce Romanoski; and to M. Russell Buchanan, M.A., M.L.S., who assisted us with the preparation of the index.

Finally, we extend our sincere gratitude to our families and our colleagues at Thomas Jefferson University and Temple University, College of Allied Health, Department of Physical Therapy for their support and encouragement throughout the writing of this text.

L.E.B.
D.A.N.

Contributors

Lorraine E. Buchanan, R.N. M.S.N.
SCI Project Coordinator, Regional SCI Center of Delaware Valley, Thomas Jefferson University, Philadelphia, Pennsylvania

Barbara E. Brown, B.S., O.T.R.
Director of Occupational Therapy, Woodrow Wilson Rehabilitation Center, Fishersville, Virginia

Helen M. Cioshi, C.R.N.P., M.S.N., C.R.R.N.
Clinical Coordinator of SCI Follow-up Systems, Regional SCI Center of Delaware Valley, Magee Rehabilitation Hospital, Philadelphia, Pennsylvania

John F. Ditunno, Jr., M.D.
SCI Project Director, Regional SCI Center of Delaware Valley, Professor and Chairman, Department of Rehabilitation Medicine, Thomas Jefferson University, Philadelphia, Pennsylvania

Page Duncanson, B.S., O.T.R.
Occupational Therapy Department, Johnston-Willis Hospital, Richmond, Virginia
formerly:
Clinical Education Supervisor, Occupational Therapy Department, Woodrow Wilson Rehabilitation Center, Fishersville, Virginia

Cynthia L. Kraft, R.N., M.S., C.R.R.N.
Liaison Nurse, Regional SCI Center of Delaware Valley, Magee Rehabilitation Hospital, Philadelphia, Pennsylvania

Scott A. Mackler, M.D., Ph.D.
Department of Medicine, University Hospital, Boston University, Boston, Massachusetts
formerly of:
Department of Anatomy, David Mahoney Institute of Neurological Sciences, University of Pennsylvania, Philadelphia, Pennsylvania

Deborah A. Nawoczenski, M.Ed., P.T.
Assistant Professor, Department of Physical Therapy, College of Allied Health Professions, Temple University, Philadelphia, Pennsylvania

Dean Ragone, B.A.
Haddonfield, New Jersey

Cathy Redd, Ph.D.
Director of Psychology, Magee Rehabilitation Hospital, Philadelphia, Pennsylvania

Margaret E. Rinehart, M.S., P.T.
Instructor in Physical Therapy, Thomas Jefferson University, College of Allied Health Sciences, Philadelphia, Pennsylvania

William E. Staas, Jr., M.D.
Co-Associate Director for On-Going Care, Regional SCI Center of Delaware Valley, President and Medical Director, Magee Rehabilitation Hospital, Philadelphia, Pennsylvania

Michael Selzer, M.D., Ph.D.
Department of Neurology, David Mahoney Institute of Neurological Sciences, University of Pennsylvania, Philadelphia, Pennsylvania

Byron Woodbury, Ph.D.
Director of Clinical Service, Department of Psychology, St. Lawrence Rehabilitation Center, Lawrenceville, New Jersey

Contents

CHAPTER 1

An Overview

LORRAINE E. BUCHANAN, R.N., M.S.N.

Traumatic spinal cord injury (SCI) is a devastating challenge for the injured individual, for family and friends, for the health care community, and for society as a whole. All concerned members of the health care and lay communities must address this problem by a concerted effort.

The increased survival rate for persons with traumatic spinal cord injury makes this multidisciplinary problem even more important. Although the medical issues of the emergency and acute phases remain of paramount importance, rehabilitation and societal issues now arise routinely as increasing numbers of persons with spinal cord injuries return to community living.

The scope of the problem of SCI can be measured in terms of incidence, dollar costs, and revenue and productivity losses to society. It can also be measured in terms of issues specific to each individual, such as chronic illness, repeated acute illness, loss of independence, emotional and social maladjustment, income losses and financial stresses, and overall quality of life concerns.

It is important that each member of the multidisciplinary allied health team appreciate the full scope of the problem for society and for the individual, as well as understand his or her own role within a defined management approach.

This chapter sets the stage for this book by briefly reviewing the anatomy of the spine and spinal cord and describing the neuropathologic processes of spinal cord injury. In addition, a review of incidence, prevalence, and the demographics of the SCI population is presented. Management approaches and more specific issues are addressed in subsequent chapters.

Anatomy of the Spine and Spinal Cord

SPINE

The spine, or vertebral column, is comprised of vertebral bodies separated by intervertebral disks. A flexible column, it is situated in the midline and forms the posterior portion of the trunk. For the sake of nomenclature, the vertebral column is divided into *cervical, thoracic, lumbar, sacral,* and *coccygeal* regions.

Viewed laterally, the vertebral column can be seen as a series of curves—the anteriorly convex *cervical curve,* the concave *thoracic curve,* the convex *lumbar curve,* and the concave *pelvic curve* (Fig. 1.1).

There are 7 cervical vertebrae (C1–7), 12 thoracic vertebrae (T1–12), 5 lumbar vertebrae (L1–5), 5 fused sacral vertebrae (S1–S5), and 4 fused coccygeal vertebrae. The cervical, thoracic, and lumbar vertebrae are regarded as true or movable vertebrae because they are not fused in the mature adult as are the sacral and coccygeal vertebrae.

A typical vertebra is comprised of an anterior portion, the *vertebral body,* and a posterior portion, the *neural arch.* The neural arch consists

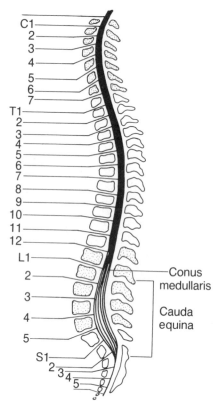

C1
2
3
4
5
6
7
T1
2
3
4
5
6
7
8
9
10
11
12
L1
2
3
4
5
S1
2
3
4
5

Conus
medullaris

Cauda
equina

Figure 1.1. Vertebral column.

of a pair of anterolateral *pedicles*, a pair of posterolateral *laminae*, four *articular processes*, two *transverse processes*, and one *spinous process* (Fig. 1.2).

The cervical vertebrae are the smallest of the movable vertebrae. They can be distinguished from the thoracic and lumbar vertebrae by the presence of a foramen in each transverse process that allows passage of the vertebral artery and accompanying plexuses of the vertebral vein and sympathetic nerves.

The thoracic vertebrae are of intermediate size and increase in size from T1 to T12. They differ from the vertebrae of other regions by the presence of *demifacets* on the lateral portions of the vertebral bodies that articulate with the ribs. The vertebral bodies of the thoracic region are heart-shaped, and the long spinous processes project inferiorly.

The lumbar vertebrae are particularly large and heavy and are distinguished from other vertebrae by the presence of accessory and *mammillary processes*. The sacrum is triangular in appearance, and its central portion consists of the fused bodies of the sacral vertebrae.

There are structural variations in the first cervical, thoracic, fifth lumbar, and first sacral vertebrae that represent adaptations necessary for joining the vertebral column with adjacent structures. In addition, there are differences in the vertebral structure at the junctions of the

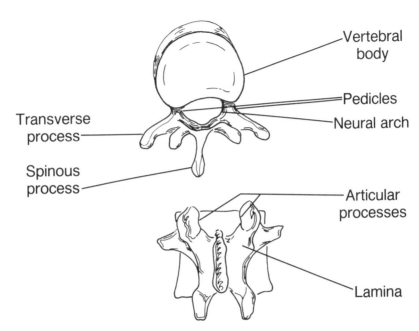

Figure 1.2.   Typical vertebra.

cervicothoracic, thoracolumbar and lumbosacral vertebrae. The vertebrae at these junctions are called *transitional vertebrae* and possess characteristics common to both regions.

The *spinal canal*, or vertebral foramen, is formed by the junction of the vertebral body and the neural arch; successive vertebral foramina form the vertebral canal. In the cervical and lumbar regions of the vertebral column, the spinal canal is large and triangular. In the thoracic region, where freedom of motion is more limited, the spinal canal is small and rounded because no plexuses arise from this area.

The supporting structures that give the spine stability include the *anterior longitudinal ligament*, the *posterior longitudinal ligament*, the *intervertebral disks*, and the musculature of the neck and trunk. Further stability is provided for the vertebral column by the *ligamenta flava*, the *supraspinal ligament*, the *ligamentum nuchae*, the *interspinal ligament*, and the *intertransverse ligament* (Fig. 1.3).

The anterior longitudinal ligament is a strong, broad band of fibers that extends from the *axis* (C2) to the sacrum along the anterior surfaces of the vertebral bodies. It adheres to the intervertebral disks and the prominent margins of the vertebral bodies.

The posterior longitudinal ligament, located within the spinal canal, extends from the axis (C2) to the sacrum, thinning as it descends along the posterior surfaces of the vertebral bodies. It also adheres to the intervertebral disks and the prominent surfaces of the vertebral bodies.

The primary connection between the vertebral bodies is provided by the intervertebral disks. The size and shape of the intervertebral disks correspond to the vertebral bodies with which they articulate,

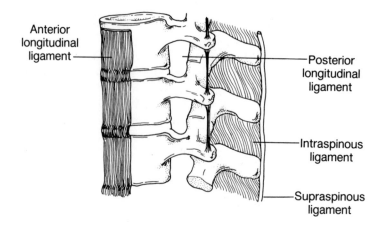

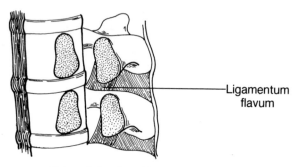

Figure 1.3. Spinal ligaments.

except in the cervical region where they are smaller than the adjacent vertebrae. The intervertebral disks are adherent to the thin layers of hyaline cartilage that cover the surfaces of the vertebral bodies.

The circumference of the intervertebral disk is comprised of fibrocartilage, and the center contains a mucoid material in which collagen fibers are embedded. This central *nucleus pulposus* is especially well developed in the lumbar region. The intervertebral disks serve a primary function as articular shock absorbers for the vertebral column.

MOVEMENT OF THE SPINE

The amount of motion that is possible in the spine is determined by the size of the intervertebral disks. The direction of motion is determined by the orientation of the facet joints. The orientation of the facet joint surfaces varies from region to region, and the predominant motion that occurs in each region depends upon the plane of facet orientation.

The motions of flexion and extension, and of lateral flexion and rotation, occur with a greater range of lateral flexion and rotation in the cervical region than in any other region of the spine. The *maximum bending moment* in flexion and extension occurs between C4 and C6. Therefore, this is the location of the majority of cervical spine injuries.

The thoracic region is less flexible and more stable than the cervical region because of the limitations imposed by the ribs, spinous processes, and joint capsules in this region. All motions are possible, but they are restricted according to the changes in the facet orientation from the upper to lower thoracic region. Flexion and extension are limited in the upper thoracic spine, but increase in the lower thoracic spine. Rotation is not limited in the upper thoracic spine, but becomes more restricted in the lower thoracic spine.

The lumbar facets favor flexion and extension and limit lateral flexion and rotation. Flexion is more limited in the lumbar spine than extension. Lateral flexion and rotation progressively diminish in the lower region of the lumbo sacral spine.

The ability of the spine to resist an imposed load—stiffness—is determined by the design of the facet joints. The spine becomes increasingly stiffer from T7 to L4, with a peak at T12 to L1. It is at this level that the facet joints hinder rotation by their change in position. This is a level of high stress concentration and is subject to mechanical failure, as evidenced by the high incidence of spine injury at the thoraco lumbar junction. Anatomically, this articulation may vary among individuals from T9 to L1.

SPINAL CORD

The spinal cord is a discrete, cylindrical mass of nerve tissue contained within the spinal canal. Until the end of the first trimester of embryonic development, the spinal cord is continuous with the full length of the spinal canal. After the first trimester, the vertebral column grows much faster in length than the spinal cord.

As a result, the adult spinal cord ends at the upper border of the second lumbar vertebra (although anatomical differences occur), where it tapers to form the *conus medullaris*. A meningeal sheath, the *filum terminale* arises from this cone-shaped termination of the spinal cord and anchors it to the dorsal surface of the coccyx. The spinal cord can be divided into *cervical, thoracic, lumbar, sacral, and coccygeal* regions according to the segmental nature of spinal nerves originating from it.

MENINGES

The spinal cord is surrounded by three membranes, which are collectively referred to as *meninges*: the *dura mater*, the *arachnoid*, and the *pia mater*. The *epidural space* separates the dura mater from the vertebral column, the *subdural space* separates the dura mater from the arachnoid membranes, and the *subarachnoid space* separates the arachnoid from the pia mater membranes. The pia mater is adherent to the surface of the spinal cord. Cerebrospinal fluid (CSF) is contained within the subarachnoid space (Fig. 1.4).

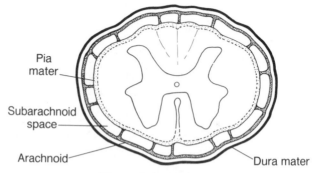

Figure 1.4.   Meninges.

ENLARGEMENTS

The spinal cord has two major levels of enlargement that correspond to the attachments of groups of nerves (large peripheral nerve plexuses). The *cervical enlargement* extends from C5 to T1 and marks the origin of the nerves for the upper extremities (brachial plexus), whereas the *lumbar enlargement* extends from L1 to S4 and marks the origins of the lower extremity nerves (lumbar plexus).

SPINAL NERVES

There are 31 pairs of spinal nerves that arise from the spinal cord at each level and exit through the intervertebral foramina. Each nerve has an *anterior* or motor *root* (or ventral root) comprised primarily of motor fibers and a *posterior* or sensory *root* (or dorsal root) that is primarily comprised of sensory fibers.

Each dorsal (sensory) root contains an aggregation of sensory nerve cell bodies at the level of the intervertebral foramen that is known as the *dorsal root ganglion*. The cell bodies of the ventral (motor) nerve roots are located in the anterior horn of the gray matter and are known as the *anterior horn cells*. Each corresponding anterior and dorsal root joins distal to the dorsal root ganglion and forms a mixed (motor and sensory) spinal nerve (Fig. 1.5).

There are 8 cervical, 12 thoracic, 5 lumbar, 5 sacral, and 1 coccygeal nerve. In the cervical region, the spinal nerve roots exit the spinal canal above the level of their corresponding vertebrae. However, the eighth cervical spinal nerve root exits below the level of the C7 vertebra, and below this level, all spinal nerve roots exit below the level of the corresponding vertebrae.

The difference in growth rate accounts for the fact that the spinal cord segments are located above their corresponding vertebral levels. Therefore, the lower the cord segment, the longer the distance between the origin of the spinal nerve root and its exit from the spinal canal.

The spinal nerve roots of the lumbar and sacral areas must travel the greatest distance from their cord origin to exit from the canal. At these levels the spinal nerve roots are not bundled and are known collectively as the *cauda equina* because of their similarity in appearance to a horse's tail.

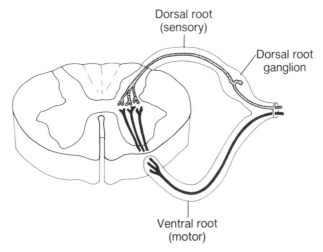

Figure I.5. Dorsal and ventral spinal nerve roots.

GRAY AND WHITE MATTER

The central nervous system (CNS) is comprised primarily of two types of nerve tissue. The *gray matter* contains the cell bodies of the neurons and their dendrites. It varies in shape, size, and appearance at different levels of the spinal cord. There is a greater amount of gray matter to white matter in the cervical and lumbar enlargements. The *white matter* is composed of bundles of nerve fibers, primarily myelinated axons.

In cross-section, the spinal cord is divided into symmetrical lateral halves by the *anterior median fissure* and the *posterior median sulcus*. The anterior median fissure is deep and contains a fold of pia mater. The posterior median sulcus is a shallow groove.

Gray matter is located centrally, forming an "H" or butterfly shape. White matter surrounds the central gray and is divided into *funiculi* or large bundles of fibers (also called columns). There are three columns or *funiculi* of white matter—anterior, lateral, and posterior (Fig. 1.6).

The anterior column contains the descending (motor) tracts— *ventral corticospinal, vestibulospinal, tectospinal,* and *reticulospinal*— as well as the ascending (sensory) tracts—*ventral spinothalamic* and *spino-olivary.* The primary functions mediated by these tracts include motor function, posture reflexes, light touch, and pressure.

The lateral white column contains the descending (motor) tracts— *lateral corticospinal, rubrospinal,* and *olivospinal.* The ascending (sensory) tracts contained within the lateral white matter include the *dorsal spinocerebellar,* the *ventral spinocerebellar,* and the *lateral spinothalamic.* The primary functions mediated by the tracts of the lateral white column include subconscious proprioception for control of locomotion, pain, temperature, and motor function.

The posterior white column, or dorsal column, contains the *fasciculus interfascicularis* descending (motor) tract and the *fasciculus gracilis* and the *fasciculus cuneatus* ascending (sensory) tracts. The

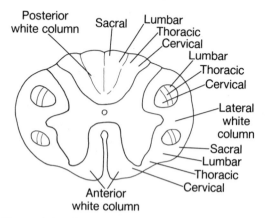

Figure 1.6.   Cross-sectional view of the spinal cord.

posterior column also contains small bundles of afferent fibers that interconnect various spinal cord levels. Also serving this function, the *fasciculus proprius* is present in all three white columns surrounding the central gray matter. The dorsal column mediates proprioception, vibration, two-point discrimination, deep pressure, and touch.

In general, the primary motor tracts are located in the anterior and anterolateral portion of the spinal cord, and the primary sensory tracts are located in the posterior and posterolateral portions. This is an important generalization, as it provides an understanding of the clinical symptoms that may be present in an incomplete lesion of the spinal cord.

CENTRAL CANAL

The *central canal* runs the full length of the spinal cord from the fourth ventricle in the medulla oblongata to the end of the conus medullaris. It contains CSF and is lined with ependymal cells.

NEURON

The *neuron* is the basic morphologic and functional unit of the nervous system. It is comprised of a cell body, a single axon, and dendritic processes (Fig. 1.7). Within the CNS, a single nerve tract is made up of a single neuron or a series of neurons that communicate with each other, i.e., transmit nerve impulses via chemical synaptic connections.

Neurons that transmit motor impulses and are contained within the CNS are called *upper motor neurons*. Motor neurons whose cell bodies are located in the spinal cord and whose axons exit the spinal cord to innervate skeletal muscle are called *lower motor neurons*.

Clinically, it is important to differentiate between upper motor neuron and lower motor neuron lesions. Upper motor neuron lesions result in spastic paralysis because of the sparing of injury to the lower motor neuron reflex arcs. Lower motor neuron lesions result in flaccid paralysis. Injuries to the spinal cord at the level of the conus medullaris and the cauda equina are lower motor neuron lesions.

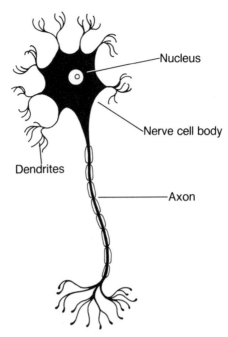

Figure 1.7.   Neuron.

REFLEX ARC

Reflexes are mediated in the spinal cord and require no cerebral intervention. The reflex arc is comprised of an efferent (motor) neuron, a receptor, an afferent (sensory) neuron, and an intercalated neuron that relays the impulse from the afferent to the efferent neuron.

DERMATOMES

The area of the skin that is innervated by a single dorsal spinal nerve is called a *dermatome*. The entire cutaneous surface of the body has been mapped out by numerous researchers over the years. However, there is some disagreement over the specific dermatomal segmentation in some areas, i.e., the specific dermatomes of C4 and C5 in the clavicular area. The dermatomal segmentation of the trunk is particularly important because there are no functional components upon which to base the assessment of neurologic level in this area.

The Physical Problem

Neurologic deficit occurs when sufficient force is exerted on the spinal cord. The force exerted on the cord may take the form of an immediate physical alteration of the structures of the cord, such as is seen with a wound caused by a missile, foreign body, or intraspinal mass such as a bone fragment that actually pierces the spinal cord and anatomically severs some or all of the neural components. Often, however, the spinal cord remains intact. That is, the neural components remain physically contiguous, but the spinal cord undergoes a delayed autodestructive process that was initiated by the force.

Immediate destruction of the spinal cord by physically severing the neural elements is clear: Nerve connections cannot function if they are anatomically separated. However, the destruction that results from the delayed autodestructive process requires further explanation.

The autodestructive process following blunt force injury to the spinal cord is a process involving (a) immediate concussion of the neural elements of the spinal cord, (b) microhemorrhaging of the central gray matter vessels, (c) edema of the spinal cord secondary to the hemorrhagic process, and (d) resultant necrosis of the spinal cord tissue.

The necrotic process has been demonstrated experimentally to consume 40% of the cross-sectional cord at the level of injury within 4 hours of trauma. Seventy percent of the cord may be destroyed within 24 hr. Once the process is complete, the necrotic area includes 100% of the cross-sectional level of the cord and extends several millimeters superior and inferior to the injured level, forming a football-shaped lesion. Understanding the delayed, autodestructive pathophysiology of spinal cord injury is important in the early phases of care and is addressed in the subsequent chapters on emergency and acute phase management approaches.

Neurologic deficit resulting from spinal cord injury may or may not be accompanied by concomitant injury to the vertebral column and other musculoskeletal structures that surround the spinal cord. The severity of the neurologic deficit depends upon both the extent and the level of the spinal cord injury.

EXTENT OF INJURY

The *extent* of the injury describes whether the lesion is *complete* or *incomplete*. A complete spinal cord injury is one in which all motor and sensory function is lost below the level of the injury.

Complete Spinal Cord Injury.   At the time of complete injury, all motor power, sensation, and reflexes are lost in those areas of the extremities and trunk that are mediated by the spinal nerves at and below the level of the injured cord. Flaccid paralysis occurs immediately and lasts throughout the initial phase of neurogenic shock (also known as *spinal shock*).

In upper motor neuron lesions the resolution of spinal shock is determined by the return of deep-tendon reflexes. This may occur hours or weeks after the injury. There is a concomitant loss of visceral function, including flaccid paralysis of the bowel and bladder. When spinal shock subsides, the flaccid paralysis is replaced by spasticity when the level of the cord injury is above the level of conus medullaris. As previously mentioned, if the injury is at or below the conus medullaris (lower motor neuron lesions), the paralysis of skeletal and visceral musculature remains flaccid.

Incomplete Spinal Cord Injury.   If there is any function intact below the level of injury, the lesion is incomplete by definition. There are four major incomplete spinal cord syndromes. They can be differentiated by the clinical symptoms presented, and each reflects the areas of the spinal cord predominantly affected by the injury.

An *anterior cord syndrome* results primarily in a profound motor loss below the level of injury. Destruction of the anterior portions of the white and gray matter of the spinal cord affects the major corticospinal (motor) tracts and, to a lesser extent, the sensory tracts that mediate light touch and pressure (Fig. 1.8A).

Conversely, a *posterior cord syndrome* results primarily in a loss of sensory function below the level of injury. Major motor tracts in the anterior portion of the spinal cord may be largely unaffected, whereas the sensory modalities of proprioception, discrimination, and vibration are severely impaired or lost (Fig. 1.8B).

In a *central cord injury*, the neural elements of the upper extremities are more severely impaired than are those of the lower extremities when the pathophysiologic process is primarily limited to the central portions of the gray and white matter of the spinal cord (Fig. 1.8C). Upper extremity function is mediated by the medial corticospinal tracts in the cord. Therefore, motor and sensory function in the lower extremities may be affected, but to a lesser extent than in the upper extremities. Central cord injury is a fairly common occurrence in individuals who have congenitally narrow spinal canals and in those in whom concomitant osteoarthritic changes have caused a narrowing of the spinal canal. For this reason, elderly persons are particularly susceptible to central cord injury

A *Brown-Sequard syndrome* results from an anterior-posterior hemisection of the spinal cord (Fig. 1.8D). It is primarily caused by a penetrating wound in which the foreign body or missile severs virtually half the neural elements of the spinal cord. When the elements

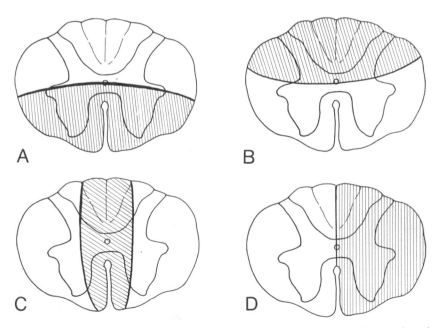

Figure 1.8. *A,* Anterior cord syndrome. *B,* Posterior cord syndrome. *C,* central cord syndrome. *D,* Brown-Sequard syndrome.

of only one lateral portion of the spinal cord are destroyed, the loss of both motor and sensory function occurs below the level of the injury. There is a characteristic loss of motor function, deep touch, proprioception, and vibration on the ipsilateral side below the lesion, with a loss of pain, temperature, simple touch, and pressure on the contralateral side of the body.

The descending motor tracts of the spinal cord cross to the opposite side at the level of the medulla oblongata—the *decussation of the pyramids.* The ascending sensory tracts cross to the opposite side at or about the level in which the dorsal roots enter the cord. This explains the somewhat ironic pattern of neurologic loss in a Brown-Sequard syndrome.

An incomplete spinal cord lesion may present symptoms that are clearly characteristic of one of the four syndromes described above; it may involve a combination of syndromes, such as a mixed central cord/Brown-Sequard syndrome; or it may only involve partial symptoms of a particular syndrome. Incomplete spinal cord injuries may also be functionally classified according to the *Frankel Scale* system (Table 1.1).

LEVEL OF INJURY

The severity of the loss is determined by the level at which the injury occurs. Each level of the spinal cord innervates specific motor and sensory functions. Therefore, the higher the level of lesion, the more profound is the loss of function.

Quadriplegia results when an injury occurs to the spinal cord in the cervical region (between C1 and T1). The term "quadriplegia" refers to paralysis of all four extremities (complete spinal cord injury). *Paraplegia* refers to paralysis of the lower extremities and results from an injury to the spinal cord in the thoracic, lumbar, sacral, or coccygeal areas of the spine. The terms "quadraparesis" and "paraparesis" refer

Table 1.1
Frankel Scale Functional Classification[a]

A **COMPLETE**
    No preservation of motor or sensory function
B **INCOMPLETE—PRESERVED SENSATION ONLY**
    Preservation of any sensation below the level of injury, except phantom sensations
C **INCOMPLETE—PRESERVED MOTOR NONFUNCTIONAL**
    Preserved motor function without useful purpose; sensory function may or may not be preserved
D **INCOMPLETE—PRESERVED MOTOR FUNCTIONAL**
    Preserved functional voluntary motor function that is functionally useful
E **COMPLETE RECOVERY**
    Complete return of all motor and sensory function, but may still have abnormal reflexes

[a] From "Standards for Neurological Classification Of Spinal Injury Patients," American Spinal Injury Association, November 1983.

to weakness, rather than total paralysis, and may be used when an injury is incomplete.

The diaphragm is innervated by the phrenic nerve primarily via the C3–5 spinal nerves. Any injury to the spinal cord above the level of C4 may render the individual incapable of spontaneous, independent breathing. It also causes a loss of all voluntary control of all extremity and trunk musculature, as well as a loss of all sensation below the level of injury. If the C4 spinal nerve is undamaged, diaphragmatic function may be intact, and the individual may be capable of independent abdominal breathing.

At each successive lower level of the spinal cord, innervation to the muscles of the upper extremities, trunk, and lower extremities is spared sequentially. The motor innervation, by level, is described in Table 1.2. The functional significance of each level of injury is described in Table 7.2.

There may be a *zone of injury* of up to three neurologic levels below the level of complete injury where there may be some preservation of function. This zone of injury does not negate the diagnosis of complete spinal cord injury.

Classification of Neurologic Level.   Consistent classification of the level of spinal cord injury is important in the communication and understanding of the clinical significance of the injury.

Traditionally, each medical and surgical discipline has applied its own interest and expertise to level classification. For example, the orthopedic surgeon may classify the injury by the level of bony injury, the neurosurgeon may refer to the injured level of the cord, and the rehabilitation medicine physician may classify the injury according to the spared functional level. In many instances, there may be three different level classifications in a single patient. Needless to say, great confusion may occur.

Table 1.2
Motor Level Classification[a]

Spinal Nerve	Muscle(s)	Function
C4	Diaphragm/trapezius	Shoulder shrug
C5	Deltoid/biceps	Elbow flexion
C6	Wrist extensors	Wrist dorsiflexion
C7	Triceps	Elbow extension
C8	Flexor profundus	Finger flexion
T1	Hand intrinsics	Finger abduction, finger adduction
T2–L1	Use sensory level	
L2	Iliopsoas	
L3	Quadriceps	
L4	Tibialis anterior	
L5	Extensor hallucis longus	
S1	Gastrocnemius	
S2–S5	Use sensory level	

[a] Adapted from "Standards For Neurological Classification Of Spinal Injury Patients," American Spinal Injury Association, November 1983.

In 1983, the American Spinal Injury Association (ASIA) developed standards for neurologic classification of spinal injury patients in an attempt to minimize the difficulties that result from misclassification and miscommunication. The basic premise of the ASIA standards is that the level of injury is the lowest level in which functional motor power and sensation remain intact after spinal cord injury. Functional motor power is described as a manual muscle test score of ⅗ or greater, when ⅗ is equivalent to the ability to accomplish full range of motion against gravity, but without resistance.

Clinical Effects of Traumatic Spinal Cord Injury

As previously stated, the immediate effects of complete spinal cord injury include a total loss of motor and sensory function below the level of injury to the spinal cord. Other symptoms that should be recognized include:

1. Neurogenic (spinal) shock evidence by marked hypotension, brady-cardia, and loss of reflexes;
2. Flaccid paralysis of the bladder with urinary retention;
3. Flaccid paralysis of the bowel with paralytic ileus;
4. Loss of perspiration below the level of injury,

Traumatic spinal cord injury has profound lasting effects on vir-tually every system of the body (Table 1.3). The problems experienced in each area and the recommended management approaches are addressed in detail in the remainder of this text.

Incidence/Prevalence

Estimates of incidence of traumatic spinal cord injury have ranged from 20 per million to 60 per million of population each year. Although several states have established spinal cord injury (SCI) registries in recent years, spinal cord injury is not a reportable injury, and there-fore, actual incidence figures are not known. It is estimated, however, that there are between 7,000 and 10,000 new cases of traumatic spinal cord injury each year in the United States.

Prevalence is estimated to be well over 200,000 in the United States. The improved management approaches that have been devel-

Table 1.3
Systems Compromised in Spinal Cord Injury

Cardiovascular
Integumentary
Gastrointestinal
Genitourinary
Metabolic
Neuromusculoskeletal
Psychosocial/sexual
Respiratory
Vocational

oped, implemented, and documented by the federally designated Model Spinal Cord Injury System Program since 1972 have demonstrated that the survival rate for persons with traumatic SCI can be significantly increased. As a result, it can be anticipated that the prevalence will continue to increase as greater numbers of persons return to community living.

Characteristics of the Spinal Cord Injury Population

ETIOLOGY

Although the many causes of traumatic SCI may vary by region, the most common causes, in decreasing order of magnitude, are vehicular accidents, falls, gunshot wounds, and diving accidents. Other causes include accidents resulting from persons being hit by falling objects, sports-related incidents (football, rugby, swimming, horseback riding, etc.), penetrating wounds other than gunshot wounds, medical-surgical misadventures, and other miscellaneous events (Table 1.4).

Automobile accidents account for over 40% of all spinal cord injuries. In the past several years, accident prevention efforts directed toward promoting the use of seatbelts and discouraging driving while intoxicated seem to be having some effect on reducing the number of automobile related injuries in some areas of the country. It can be anticipated that this reduction will continue as more states enact mandatory seatbelt legislation and enforce stricter drunk driving laws.

Accidents happen, however, and although many can be prevented with caution and forethought, others appear to be unavoidable. Falls occur in the home, on the job, and in the community. Spinal cord injuries resulting from gunshot wounds, stab wounds, and other acts of violence are difficult to prevent; indeed, there are existing laws that are designed to prevent such incidents!

The incidence of sports-related injuries has markedly decreased

Table 1.4
Etiology of Spinal Cord Injury[a]

Motor vehicle accidents		47.7%
Falls		20.8%
Acts of violence		14.6%
Sports		14.2%
Diving	66.0%	
Football	6.1%	
Snow skiing	3.8%	
Surfing	3.1%	
Trampoline	2.6%	
Wrestling	2.3%	
Gymnastics	2.2%	
Horseback	2.0%	
Other sports	11.9%	
Other		2.7%

[a] From *Spinal Cord Injury: Facts & Figures*, Birmingham, AL, National Spinal Cord Injury Statistical Center, 1986.

in recent years. Specifically, football injuries, which once occurred with alarming predictability each fall, have been minimized with the enforcement of regulations that strictly prohibit the use of certain tackling techniques, such as "spearing." Safety equipment has also been developed in attempts to apply a technological approach to the prevention of disabling injuries.

The one major cause of traumatic spinal cord injury that is preventable in virtually every case is diving. The overwhelming majority of diving-related spinal cord injuries occur when people dive into water that is less than 4 to 6 feet deep. The American Red Cross recommends that water must be 12 to 14 feet deep before it is safe for diving.

In some cases, the depth of the water is not known, as may occur when diving into an unsupervised lake, pond, or stream. In other cases, the depth may be known to the individual, but the danger of diving into shallow water was not considered, as happens when diving into an above-ground pool or the shallow end of an in-ground pool.

Unfortunately, spinal cord injuries also occur when people dive from a diving board into an in-ground pool that has a steep slope from the supposedly "safe" deep end to the shallow end. Because of the person's trajectory off the board, the water may only be 3 to 4 feet deep at the point at which the person enters the water.

It is important that the proper method of "steering up" on entering the water be employed to avoid diving-related accidents, as well as ensuring that there is sufficient water depth. Knowing how to dive is just as important as knowing where to dive.

Regardless of the cause, the best means of prevention of a spinal cord injury is consideration of the potential consequences before undertaking any physical activity. One need not avoid participating in any reasonable activity, as long as an appropriate effort is made to exercise caution, to play by the rules, to refrain from mixing alcohol or drugs with any physical activity that requires full cognitive awareness, and to avoid carelessness.

DEMOGRAPHICS

Traumatic SCI is a markedly male condition, with over 80% of all reported cases occurring in men (Table 1.5). Although there is an increasing trend of women incurring previously male-dominated illnesses, such as cardiac disease and lung cancer, that is not the case with spinal cord injury. The figures of male versus female incidence have remained virtually constant since statistics on spinal cord injury were first collected in the early 1970s.

The SCI population is also markedly young (Table 1.6). The age range is infancy to over 90 years, but over half of the SCI population

Table 1.5
Distribution by Sex

Male	82%
Female	18%

Table 1.6
Distribution by Age[a]

(yr)	(%)
0–15	4.9
16–30	61.1
31–45	19.4
46–60	9.2
61–75	4.9
76–90	1.0

[a] From *Spinal Cord Injury: Facts & Figures*, Birmingham, AL, National Spinal Cord Injury Statistical Center, 1986.

is between the ages of 15 and 30, with the most common age being 18 years. Although no age is immune, it is significantly uncommon for traumatic SCI to occur in children under the age of 14.

The racial distribution of the SCI population appears to reflect regional racial distributions. There does not appear to be a higher incidence in any particular racial or ethnic group. Marital status distribution and occupational status distribution are also consistent with societal norms for the sex and age groups that are most likely to incur spinal cord injury.

Therefore, the "average" person with SCI is male, 18 years of age, Caucasian, either a student or just starting out in the job market, single or newly married, and injured in a vehicular accident. Generalizations beyond that are very questionable. Although numerous studies have been done over the years to attempt to determine whether a particular personality type is more prone to SCI, they have not been conclusive.

An understanding of the common characteristics of the SCI population helps one appreciate the scope of the problem both to the individual and to society. Institutional and community-based programmatic planning should utilize this information to identify the resources necessary to assist this very heterogeneous population in achieving the goals of health maintenance, independence, and community living.

Suggested Readings

Carpenter M: *Human Neuroanatomy*. Baltimore, Williams & Wilkins, 1976.

Chusid JG: *Correlative Neuroanatomy and Functional Neurology*. Los Altos, CA, Lange Medical Publications, 1976.

Donovan WH, Bedbrook G: Comprehensive management of spinal cord injury. *Clinical Symposia* (Ciba) 34:2, 1982.

Ergas Z: Spinal cord injury in the United States: A statistical update. *Cen Nerv Sys Trauma* 2:19–30, 1985.

Guttman Sir L: *Spinal Cord Injuries: Comprehensive Management and Research*. London, Blackwell Scientific Publications, 1973.

Osterholm JL: *The Pathophysiology Of Spinal Cord Trauma*. Springfield, IL, Charles C Thomas, 1978.

Remington E: Diverse specialties harmonize. *JMC Alumni Bull* 30:2–7, 1981.

Spinal Cord Injury: Facts & Figures. Birmingham AL, National Spinal Cord Injury Statistical Center, 1986.

CHAPTER 2

Emergency Care

LORRAINE E. BUCHANAN, R.N., M.S.N.

A thorough knowledge of on-scene emergency spinal cord injury care is of course imperative for emergency paramedical personnel. However, it is important for every health care professional to understand the basic concepts of emergency assessment, handling, and care in the event that they are at the site of an accident before the arrival of emergency paramedical personnel.

The health care professional whose primary area of service is not in the area of emergency management should also recognize the expertise of qualified emergency paramedical personnel. The health care professional can best serve the injured individual by initiating the appropriate management before emergency personnel arrive and by assisting the emergency medical technician or paramedic after his or her arrival.

The emergency phase of care is crucial for the person with traumatic spinal cord injury. The handling—or mishandling—of the injured individual at the scene of the accident can make the difference between a lifetime of severe disability and a relatively short hospitalization with a return to able-bodied living.

As yet, no intervention has been proven capable of restoring function below the level of a complete spinal cord lesion. However, a complete injury can be worsened by mishandling if the cord is reinjured at a higher level or if the injury to the cord is not minimized to prevent the lesion from ascending and compromising higher functional levels.

An incomplete spinal cord injury can be significantly worsened by mishandling—at the scene of the accident and at any point in time before definitive spinal stabilization. It is important to remember that there is a reasonable expectation for some return of function below the level of injury for persons with incomplete lesions. Therefore, every effort must be made to maintain the incomplete nature of the injury in order to offer the injured individual the best hope for maximal recovery.

The emergency process for spinal/spinal cord injured individuals has four steps: (1) **assessment**, (2) **immobilization/stabilization**, (3) **extrication**, and (4) **transport**. These four basic steps in the emergency phase of care should be followed in sequence in all cases, unless a reasonable determination of risk to the life of the individual requires that the process be amended.

This chapter explains the rationale and concept for each step in the process and suggests methods for their implementation. No attempt is made to describe a specific intervention or particular equipment for use in all possible circumstances. Rather, it is the concept that should be learned. Improvisation, with a firm adherence to the basic concepts, should be employed in emergency situations, which can vary so greatly.

Assessment

The first goal of the assessment process is to determine the likelihood of the traumatized individual having sustained a spinal and/or spinal cord injury (SCI). An understanding of the common causes of SCI and a knowledge of the common characteristics of the SCI population provide a basis for that determination. For example, seeing a young man who was involved in an automobile accident should raise one's index of suspicion that he has suffered a spinal injury by virtue of the statistical make-up of the SCI population. Of course, further assessment is necessary to determine the exact nature of the injury.

MECHANISMS OF INJURY

The assessment process continues with an evaluation of the scene of the accident and a determination of the probable mechanism of injury. The four mechanisms that primarily result in spinal injury are hyperflexion, hyperextension, axial loading, and penetrating wounds. Each may occur alone or in combination with one or more of the others.

Hyperflexion. Normal range of motion and flexibility of the spine allow an individual to bend the spine anteriorly so that the chin can touch the chest and the hands can touch the toes. With sufficient force, any movement beyond those points can cause injury to the spine and/or spinal cord (Fig. 2.1).

Force exerted toward the anterior surface of the body or forward contact with an immovable object can create the hyperflexion mechanism. For example, when a moving car hits a tree head-on, the driver's head will continue to move forward after impact. If there is sufficient speed, the weight of the head and the force of impact cause a hyperflexion injury.

When a hyperflexion mechanism occurs, the most flexible levels of the spine act as a fulcrum with the greatest stresses created at these points. For example, in the cervical spine the greatest forward bending moment occurs at C5–6. The posterior longitudinal ligament can be stretched or torn, allowing the intervertebral disk to herniate or tear. Two or more vertebral bodies can be compressed against each other, causing fracture(s) and/or dislocation (subluxation). If the integrity of

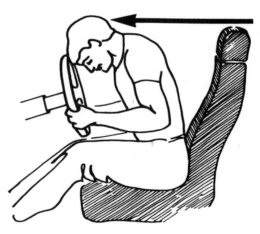

Figure 2.1.   Hyperflexion.

the spinal canal is compromised either by bone fragments or by the movement of one or more vertebral bodies, the spinal cord can be injuried. In some cases, the neural elements of the cord may be physically disrupted. In most instances, the force exerted on the spinal cord initiates the pathophysiologic process of hemorrhage, edema, and necrosis described in Chapter 1.

Hyperextension. Normal posterior range of motion of the spine allows an individual to rest the occiput on the back and to extend the dorsolumbar spine a maximum of 20° posteriorly. Any movement beyond that range is termed hyperextension and can cause injury to the bony and/or neural elements of the spine and spinal cord (Fig. 2.2).

Sufficient force exerted toward the posterior surface of the body or a rearward movement with contact with an immovable object causes hyperextension. It can also be caused when the body is hurled forward and the head strikes an object that generates a force posteriorly.

Hyperextension frequently occurs when an individual is involved in an automobile accident in which the car is rear-ended. In its mildest form, hyperextension as a result of this type of accident is commonly referred to as "whiplash." In its most severe form, it can lead to quadriplegia.

When the hyperextension mechanism occurs, the most flexible elements of the spine again act as a fulcrum. The greatest bending moment in hyperextension of the cervical spine occurs at C4–5. If there is sufficient force, the anterior longitudinal ligament can be stretched or torn, the intervertebral disk may tear or herniate, the posterior elements of the spine may compress and fracture each other, and there may be subluxation. If the integrity of the spinal canal is compromised, the neural elements of the spinal cord may be damaged. Cord damage may result from compression and/or direct trauma by bony fragments or malaligned vertebral bodies or by the pathophysiologic process of hemorrhage, edema, and necrosis initiated by the force itself.

Axial Loading (Vertical Compression). The axial loading mechanism of injury occurs when sufficient force is exerted vertically

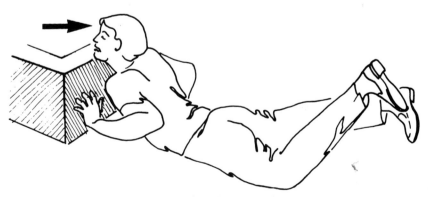

Figure 2.2. Hyperextension.

through the vertebral column. The force transferred along the spine does not in itself cause damage to the spinal cord. However, if the force is sufficient, one or more vertebral bodies absorb the intensity of the force and literally "burst." When this occurs, the vertebral body bursts in all directions—including into the spinal canal. The force of the exploding vertebral body is the force that damages the spinal cord (Fig. 2.3).

Axial loading injuries occur most frequently in cases where an individual dives head-first into shallow water, striking the top of the head on the bottom. The injury that results is usually a burst fracture of C4 or C5 with complete quadriplegia. In such cases, there is usually no concomitant demonstrable head injury; presumably, if the skull were fractured in the dive, the head would serve as a shock absorber for the cervical spine.

Axial loading injuries are also seen when a person jumps or falls from a height and lands on his or her feet. The injury that usually results is a burst fracture of T10, T11, or T12 with paraplegia. In such cases, there are often concomitant bilateral calcaneal fractures—suggesting that the impact of the heels on the ground is sufficient to cause fracture but not sufficient to minimize the vertical force on the vertebral column.

Penetrating Wounds. Low-velocity penetrating wounds and high-velocity penetrating wounds utilize two distinctly different mechanisms of injuring the spinal cord. Low-velocity penetrating wounds may be caused by stabbing in which a foreign body, such as a knife or ice pick, is manually thrust into the body or by low-velocity bullets from a small caliber handgun. High-velocity penetrating

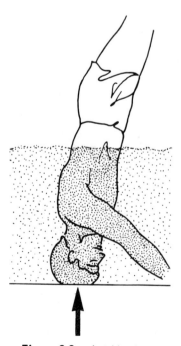

Figure 2.3. Axial loading.

wounds may be caused by bullets from high-powered rifles or by foreign bodies that are thrust into the body with great force, such as may occur when someone is injured in a explosion.

With a low-velocity penetrating wound, the mechanism of injury is usually mechanical. The missile (knife, ice pick, etc.) literally pierces the spinal cord and physically cuts the neural elements at the point of contact. There may or may not be disruption of bony elements, and stability of the vertebral column is rarely compromised, although spinal stability should still be carefully assessed.

In a high-velocity penetrating wound, the foreign body does not have to penetrate the spine or the spinal cord in order to cause damage to the neural elements. The concussive force of the missile traveling through the body can be sufficient to cause complete spinal cord injury! The concussive force alone can initiate the pathophysiologic process of hemorrhage, edema, and necrosis—without any physical disruption of the bony or neural elements of the spine or spinal cord. This is an important consideration in the assessment process.

It is very important that the emergency medical personnel determine the probable mechanisms of injury at the scene of the accident and then communicate their findings to the hospital staff. The patient may be unable to report the specifics of the accident causing the impact and injury, and the hospital personnel have no way of re-creating the accident scene to make their own determination of the mechanism of injury.

In instances where there is obvious neurologic deficit but no apparent bony injury, an understanding of the probable mechanism of injury can direct the clinical and radiographic evaluation of spinal stability. For example, in hyperextension injuries, often there is no obvious bony injury on plain film radiographs even though there is a great likelihood that severe instability of the anterior spine exists. It is possible that a dislocation of the spine may be reduced in the immobilization/extrication/transport process. With a reported probability of hyperextension, the evaluation can be directed to the anterior components of the spine and its supporting structure.

PHYSICAL ASSESSMENT

The emergency physical assessment process must, of course, begin with the evaluation of the ABCs—airway, breathing, and circulation. The initial assessment should include a measurement of blood pressure, heart rate, and respirations. If cardiopulmonary resuscitation is indicated and the initial index of suspicion is high that a spinal cord injury occurred, every effort should be made to carry out the necessary life-support measures with minimal movement of the patient's spine. This includes not hyperextending the patient's neck to open the airway, if at all possible. Instead, the chin lift or jaw thrust maneuvers should be used. The esophageal obturator airway (EOA) that is carried by many rescue units is ideal to use because it requires that the patient's neck be placed only in the neutral position for insertion of the airway.

If the blood pressure is low and the heart rate is slow, the patient is probably experiencing *neurogenic shock* and not hypovolemic shock.

Neurogenic shock occurs as a result of the sudden disruption of neurologic function, with the pooling of blood in the dependent areas of the body that results from the loss of muscle activity below the level of injury to the spinal cord. It is important to differentiate neurogenic shock from hypovolemic shock because hypovolemic shock requires immediate treatment with fluids to prevent ensuing death. Neurogenic shock should *not* be treated with the infusion of intravenous (i.v.) fluids. Indeed, treating the patient with large amounts of i.v. fluids increases the damage to the spinal cord by contributing to edema of the spinal cord. The patient with hypotension and a pulse rate under 100 who is awake, alert, oriented, and not worsening clinically should receive minimal i.v. fluids. Careful blood pressure and pulse monitoring are imperative, however.

Once the patient has been medically stabilized or when it has been established that there is no need for immediate implementation of life-support measures, the assessment of the patient should proceed methodically to ascertain the likelihood of spinal and/or spinal cord injury and associated injuries.

Assuming that the index of suspicion of spinal injury is high based on the cause and mechanism of injury, the examiner should ensure that the patient does not attempt to move until the assessment process either confirms or contradicts the suspicion. The assessment should be carried out without physically changing the position in which the injured person is found.

While providing emotional support and encouragement, the examiner should inspect the injured person's face and head for signs of obvious trauma (contusion, bulging neck vein, deviated trachea, etc.) and should ask the patient whether he or she is experiencing any pain.

The injured person should then be assessed neurologically. The simplest assessment of neurologic function is performed by determining the extent of motor function that is intact.

First, the examiner should ask the injured person if he or she is able to move the upper and lower extremities. (In cases of severe spinal cord injury, this inability may be obvious, or the injured person may volunteer that he or she cannot move.) It is important to determine whether the injury to the spinal cord is at the level of the cervical spine or below the cervical spine in order to direct subsequent care and immobilization to the appropriate area of the spine.

If the initial assessment indicates that there is a loss or diminishment of motor power, the examiner should ask the injured person to perform specific movements in order to determine the level of injury to the spinal cord. Table 2.1 describes the movements that should be assessed and the corresponding spinal cord levels indicated by normal-strength performance of each movement. For example, if the injured individual is able to breathe without assistance, can shrug the shoulders, can fully flex the elbows, but cannot dorsiflex the wrists or extend the elbows without the aid of gravity, the probable level of injury is C5.

In order to determine the extent of the injury—and to determine a probable level of injury in the thoracic spine where there is no

Table 2.1
Neuroassessment

	Motor		Sensory		Motor
C1–3	Respiration	T4	Nipple line	L2	Hip flexion
C4	Shoulder shrug	T10	Umbilicus	L3	Knee extension
C5	Elbow flexion			L4	Ankle dorsiflexion
C6	Wrist dorsiflexion			L5–S1	Knee flexion
C7	Elbow extension				
C8–T1	Fist				

voluntary functional activity to be evaluated—a sensory evaluation should be carried out. Dermatomal segmentation can be assessed. Of particular importance in level determination are the dermatomal levels that correspond to specific anatomic landmarks (and those with which most authorities agree). These include the thumbs corresponding to C6, the nipples corresponding to T4, and the umbilicus corresponding to T10.

To determine the extent of injury, a gross assessment of sensory function may be easily carried out by sticking the patient in the hands and feet with the sharp end of a pin. Although it may be difficult to assess in the field, the presence of sensation in the perineum—in the glans penis or clitoris and/or the perianal area—is indicative of an incomplete lesion when sensation is absent in all other areas below the level of injury.

If the injured person is not awake and alert enough to cooperate with a neurologic evaluation, it is best to assume that there is a high likelihood of spinal cord injury and to handle the person accordingly (if an appropriate etiology and/or mechanism of injury is also present). In the case of a cervical injury, the presence of paradoxical respirations—abdominal breathing—is a sign of cord injury. Because there is an initial loss of reflex activity below the level of injury, the unconscious person can be assessed for spinal cord injury by testing the reflexes in the lower extremities. Remember, spinal cord injury does not cause coma. Therefore, the person must be assessed for other causes of diminished level of consciousness. Handling the unconscious person as though he or she also has a spinal cord injury—by proper immobilization and careful transport—does not compromise the care that must be given for other injuries.

If the injured person does not have apparent neurologic injury but the etiology, mechanism of injury, and force of impact indicate a significant likelihood that such an injury is present, it is possible that the person may have sustained a spinal fracture or dislocation without spinal cord injury. In such cases, it is particularly important that the injured person be carefully assessed in the field and that every effort be made to ensure a comprehensive evaluation by orthopedic physicians and/or neurologists who specialize in spinal cord injury management. Vertebral injuries may become spinal cord injuries if there is spinal instability and the patient is either mishandled or allowed to move. The patient should be adequately warned about the dangers of moving (standing, walking, etc.) and strongly advised to accept medical attention.

In summary, a presumption of spinal cord injury should be made if the assessment determines that there is spinal pain or tenderness, motor power loss, and/or sensory loss—combined with the positive assessment of etiology, mechanism of injury, and patient characteristics. If the assessment is inconclusive, it is best to assume that there is injury and to handle the injured person accordingly.

Associated injuries, such as extremity fractures and head, chest, and abdominal injuries, occur in about 25% of all cases of traumatic spinal cord injury. With a loss of sensation, the pain of an extremity fracture or internal injury cannot be reported by the injured person. Therefore, the importance of a thorough physical examination cannot be minimized.

A thorough assessment is important in determining the appropriate care and handling that should be initiated in the field—but it is also extremely important in establishing the baseline for the ongoing evaluation of an injured person's neurologic status. Neurologic deficit following spinal cord trauma may fluctuate. Documentation of the baseline assessment made at the scene of the accident assists the examiner in the field and the medical/nursing staff at the receiving hospital in determining whether the patient is improving or deteriorating neurologically.

Immobilization/Stabilization

IMMOBILIZATION

Unless there is a clear threat to the injured person's safety, proper immobilization should always be carried out before extrication. Contrary to popular myth, automobiles do not often explode following collision, and unless a fire is detected, the person should be immobilized before being extricated from the damaged vehicle. In the case of diving and swimming accidents, the injured person should be immobilized before removal from the water.

The person suspected of having sustained a spinal and/or spinal cord injury should be immobilized in the position in which he or she is found—unless the neutral position is assumed naturally or can be achieved without meeting the slightest resistance or causing an exacerbation of pain or neurologic symptomatology. Although some authorities recommend that the person should always be placed in a neutral position, the author does not recommend changing the position in which the person is found *unless there is a specific reason to do so.* Appropriate reasons that would dictate patient movement include the need for life-support measures, an occluded airway that cannot be opened by alternative methods, and a predicted significant delay in securing definitive medical management.

The rationale for immobilization in the presenting position is based on common sense and an appreciation of the risk of further damage to the spinal cord. Emergency paramedical personnel in the field do not have the ability to assess radiographically the integrity of the spine. In a hospital environment, a thorough radiographic evaluation of the spine is performed in order to provide the spinal cord injury specialist with the information necessary to dictate the ways in which the patient's spine may be moved safely.

Inasmuch as emergency personnal have neither the equipment nor the expertise to carry out such a sophisticated assessment, unless there is a clear reason to change the patient's position, *do not change it*. In other words, it is most prudent to follow the old saying, "If it ain't broke, don't fix it!"

There are many different types of emergency immobilization devices commercially available. Indeed, new devices are being developed and marketed constantly. Some are better than others in preventing movement of the spine. It is not the intention of this author to advocate the usage of any particular brand of collar, spinal board, or immobilization device. However, in the following discussion, commonly used brands of equipment may be mentioned by name for the sake of illustration. It is the *concept* of immobilization that is presented here and not a review of available equipment.

During the assessment process, the patient should be encouraged not to move and should be manually immobilized. If a second rescuer is present, that person should stabilize the patient's head with his or her hands and forearms without pulling on the patient's head or neck. If a second rescuer is not present, the examiner should emphasize to the patient the importance of not moving and make every attempt to ensure compliance during the examination.

Once it is determined that the patient has likely had a spine and/ or spinal cord injury, the patient should be immobilized. If it is possible to apply a cervical collar without flexing or extending the patient's neck, do so, while taking care not to move the patient. A soft foam collar provides the least immobilization of all collars available because it permits flexion extension and rotation of the neck. A rigid custom-made collar is impractical because of the need for prefitting. The PHILADELPHIA collar or NEC-LOCK collar provide maximal support and are available in 3 to 9 sizes that can be easily applied to most patients in an emergency setting. If a collar cannot be applied, neck support should be improvised by wrapping towels or clothing around the patient's neck.

The patient should be immobilized on a rigid board before extrication. To immobilize a person seated in an automobile, first secure the patient to a short spine board (a long spinal board is placed under the short board during the extrication process). Place the short board behind the patient, fill in the spaces between the patient and the board with towels or blanket rolls, and tightly strap the patient to the board. The patient's head should be taped to the board.

If the patient is found lying on the ground, he or she should be immobilized on a long spinal board after placement of the collar. Place the board under the patient by gently "log-rolling" the patient to one side and carefully sliding *the board under the patient*. Two to four persons are needed to safely log-roll a person with spinal cord injury.

One person should stabilize the patient's head and neck, and it is this person who should direct the turning. The patient should be secured to the long spinal board with straps. The patient's head should be taped to the board with sandbags snugly placed on both sides of the patient's head and neck.

In a water rescue, the patient should be log-rolled in the water into a supine position, with the patient's head and neck supported and stabilized by the rescuer. A second rescuer should retrieve an appropriate board—either a long spinal board or a reasonable facsimile, such as a diving board, ironing board, door, etc. Regardless of the board used, the concept of immobilization should be the same: The patient should be securely stabilized on a firm surface before extrication.

It is important that the person be tightly secured on the spinal board. In the event that the patient becomes nauseated during the extrication and transport process, the patient can be turned *with* the board to prevent aspiration of vomitus. Immobilization should be adequately secure to minimize movement of or by the patient. Persons with incomplete injuries and those with upper extremity function may be capable of resisting immobilization. If patients are uncooperative, every effort must be made to maintain the immobilization and protect them from their own actions.

In summary, all persons suspected of having sustained spinal injury should be immobilized in the position in which they are found before extrication. In order to implement this concept of emergency care, paramedical personnel should be encouraged not to limit their practice to the limitations of available equipment but rather to exercise their expertise in improvisation.

STABILIZATION

Depending on the level of training, authorization, and medical support available, paramedical personnel may initiate appropriate medical stabilization measures at the scene of the accident to minimize the severity and effects of the traumatic spinal cord injury. These measures include (a) providing oxygen via mask or nasal cannula; (b) starting an i.v. with a large-bore needle and a solution of 5% dextrose and normal saline (or D5 and water) to run via a minidropper at 30 minidrops/min; (c) giving dexamethasone (Decadron) 10 mg or equivalent, one ampule of NaHCO3, cimetidine 300 mg, and Mannitol 50 i.v.; and (d) inserting a Foley catheter to straight drainage. Many paramedical rescue units are not equipped or permitted to give steroids and may not be authorized to give cimetidine and/or Mannitol or to insert a Foley catheter. However, the i.v. line should be established regardless of whether or not the medications can be given.

Medical care given to stabilize the patient at the scene of the accident should be carefully documented and reported to the hospital staff at the time of arrival.

Extrication

According to Webster's dictionary, extrication "implies the use of force or ingenuity in freeing from a difficult position or situation."

When extricating a person suspected of having sustained a spinal injury, it is ingenuity and not force that should be utilized.

If the person is appropriately immobilized, the extrication process should not be difficult. Again, it is important not to change the position of the patient, and care should be taken to maintain the immobilization and not jar the patient.

In extricating a person with suspected spinal injury from a vehicle, there may be some delay in clearing an opening large enough to remove the patient safely. Once the patient is adequately immobilized on the short spinal board or similar immobilization device, such as the KED extrication device, the patient should be placed on a long spinal board that has been inserted under the hips. If possible, pivot the patient *with the short board* and gently lower the patient onto the long spinal board. If it is not possible to insert one end of the long spinal board into the vehicle, lift the patient out of the vehicle, with adequate assistance, and place him or her onto the long board.

The most important concept in the extrication process is that it should always follow immobilization. The only rationale for extrication preceding immobilization is a clear and present danger to the life of the patient. All too often, well-meaning persons attempt to assist the victim of an accident by helping him or her to move. Paramedical and medical personnel should discourage these actions.

Transport

Transport is the final step in the emergency process in the field. It involves both the physical movement of the patient and the triage of the patient to the most appropriate acute care facility.

Once the patient has been adequately assessed, immobilized, and extricated, he or she should be transported to the nearest hospital facility that can provide the comprehensive care necessary for a person with traumatic spinal cord injury. In some instances, organizational guidelines allow for persons with suspected spinal injury to be transported directly from the scene of an accident to a Regional Spinal Cord Injury Center. In other instances, there are designated trauma centers. If neither is available nor practical based on the patient's clinical condition, the patient should be transported to the nearest emergency department (ED).

Regardless of the destination, it is important that the driver of the ambulance be advised that great speed is neither necessary nor recommended if the patient has been adequately stabilized at the scene. Even though the patient should be firmly immobilized on a spinal board, every effort should be made to avoid subjecting the patient to the physically jarring effects of such road hazards as potholes or rough road surfaces. Quick acceleration and sudden stops can also be detrimental to the person with an unstable spine injury.

During the transport, the patient should be monitored closely by the paramedical personnel. Vital signs, respiratory status, and neurologic status should be observed and recorded. Any change from the baseline assessment of clinical symptoms, neurologic deficit, heart rate, blood pressure, and respirations should be carefully noted.

Suction equipment should be readied in the event that a patient should become nauseated en route to the hospital. Suctioning minimizes the risk of aspiration. As previously mentioned, the patient may also need to be turned slightly to the side with the spinal board to prevent aspiration of vomitus.

Upon arrival at the Spinal Cord Injury Center, trauma center, or general hospital ED, the paramedical personnel should be prepared to remain with the patient long enough to ensure that the hospital staff receives complete and appropriate information regarding the assessment and care given at the scene of the accident. Rescue personnel may need to wait to retrieve their spinal board and other immobilization equipment until the patient can be safely moved to a definitive bed in the hospital. If the delay is longer than can be tolerated, arrangements should be made with the ED to "trade" equipment until the rescue squad can return.

Hospital personnel should appreciate the fact that the paramedics have carefully assessed the patient's condition and have often invested a great deal of time and effort in immobilizing the patient. It is very inappropriate for nurses and physicians to minimize the paramedic's ability to conduct an appropriate initial assessment of the patient's condition. Immobilization carefully and thoughtfully applied should not be removed before a thorough neurologic and orthopedic assessment.

Care and handling by ED personnel of the person suspected of having sustained a traumatic spinal cord injury is described in Chapter 3. Remember, comprehensive management of persons with spinal cord injury requires a continuous, organized, and systematic process from the moment of injury through lifetime follow-up. Many of the concepts and measures described in a particular phase may apply in other phases of care, depending on the needs of the individual patient.

Suggested Readings

Buchanan LE: Emergency! First aid for "spinal cord injury." *Nursing 82* 68–75, 1982.
Buchanan LE: Patient preparation and transfer to a regional spinal cord injury center. *J Neurosurg Nurs* 14:137–138, 1982.
Hughes L, Percy E: Emergency care of cervical spine injuries. *Hosp Med* 17:53, July 1981.
Kroeber MJ: Traumatic spinal injuries. *Aust Nurses' J* 45–60, 1980.

CHAPTER 3

Acute Care: Medical/Surgical Management

LORRAINE E. BUCHANAN, R.N., M.S.N.
JOHN F. DITUNNO, Jr., M.D.

Traditionally, the approach to the acute care of persons with traumatic spinal cord injury has been fragmented and limited by the general hospital's resources. Rehabilitation has often been delayed, consultations with physicians in other specialties have been avoided, and the multisystem nature of spinal cord injury has often been overlooked.

The concept of Spinal Cord Injury (SCI) Center care was first conceived and implemented by Dr. Ludwig Guttmann in England at the end of World War II. Because of the large number of Allied war-wounded persons with spinal cord injuries and the high mortality rate in the SCI population, Dr. Guttmann developed the principle of grouping SCI patients together in order to prevent many of the life-threatening complications of spinal cord injury.

Because of Dr. Guttmann's positive experience, leading spinal cord injury specialists in the United States advocated the development of regional Model System Spinal Cord Injury Centers to demonstrate the benefits of a system approach to spinal cord injury care. Through their efforts, regional centers were funded by the federal government in 1971. Each Model System SCI Center is designed to meet five basic criteria: (1) a system of emergency care and early referral; (2) coordination of acute medical/surgical care; (3) rehabilitation management beginning at the onset of acute care; (4) vocational evaluation, counseling, and placement; and (5) a system of lifetime follow-up care.

This chapter describes the coordination of acute medical/surgical care for persons with spinal cord injury as demonstrated by the Model System SCI Centers in the United States. Each Model System SCI Center meets the comprehensive needs of the SCI patient by utilizing a multidisciplinary, system approach and the unique resources of its own program.

In the following discussion the traditional, fragmented, nonsystem approach to care is only mentioned to highlight its deficiencies. Many patients, however, are still cared for in community hospitals. Therefore, this chapter stresses the concepts of acute care, rather than the role relationships, facilities, and resources that are necessary to provide comprehensive system care. It is important to remember, however, that the utilization of a coordinated team approach is essential to address adequately the many needs of the person with traumatic spinal cord injury, regardless of the institutional setting.

Initial Care in the Emergency Department

The principles of emergency care at the scene of the accident were presented in Chapter 2. Once the patient suspected of having sustained a traumatic SCI arrives at the hospital emergency department (ED), three of the four steps of the emergency process—assessment, immobilization/stabilization, and transport—must be repeated.

ASSESSMENT PROCESS

The first step in the assessment process in the ED requires direct communication with the paramedical personnel who accompany the patient. A complete history of events should be received, including the cause and probable mechanism of injury, a report of the paramedic's clinical findings at the time of arrival at the accident scene, a summary report of any changes in the patient's clinical or neurologic status since the time of initial assessment, a description of the immobilization techniques employed, a report of any difficulties encountered in the extrication and transfer process, and a complete report of all medical care given at the scene and enroute to the hospital. Care should also be taken to secure a written report of the paramedic's activities to ensure appropriate communication with the entire team.

Direct patient assessment should occur simultaneously with communication with paramedical personnel. Again, assessment must begin with the "ABCs." If life-support measures are indicated, appropriate support may be required from the anesthesia department for nasotracheal or endotracheal intubation using fiberoptic technology and from respiratory therapy for ventilation support and monitoring of respiratory parameters.

Every effort should be made to perform cardiopulmonary resuscitation without changing the patient's position or removing the immobilization applied in the field, if at all possible. If the patient has sustained a spine or spinal cord injury, resuscitation efforts can cause or increase the neurologic deficits, and anything that can be done to minimize the possibility of further trauma is of great importance. However, life—and not function—is the paramount issue.

Once it has been established that emergency life-support measures are not indicated or once the patient's medical condition has been stabilized, the full assessment process should begin. The following areas must be thoroughly assessed by the ED and SCI team (or trauma team) personnel:

1. Neurologic level and extent of injury;
2. Orthopedic injuries of the vertebral column;
3. Respiratory compromise secondary to neurologic injury or associated chest injury;
4. Cardiovascular compromise secondary to neurologic injury or associated chest injury;
5. Gastrointestinal compromise secondary to neurologic injury or associated abdominal injury;
6. Genitourinary compromise secondary to neurologic injury or associated abdominal or genitalia injury;
7. Associated injuries of the head, chest, abdomen, and extremities;
8. Significant medical history.

A detailed neurologic examination should be performed by a physician experienced in spinal cord injury. The neurologic level and extent of injury should be carefully documented. Table 3.1 presents an example of a form that can be utilized to document a complete neurologic examination. Whenever possible, two experienced examiners should examine the patient independently to reduce the possibility of error in the neurologic evaluation.

The basic components of the neurologic evaluation are a deter-

Table 3.1

REGIONAL SPINAL CORD INJURY CENTER NEUROLOGICAL EXAMINATION PAGE ONE	ADDRESSOGRAPH

____ Pre-admission to center   ____ Transfer to Rehab

____ Admission to Center   ____ Rehab Discharge

____ Pre-operative   ____ Follow-up

____ Post-operative   ____ Other

MOTOR

Check the strength grade of the following muscles:

Root	Muscle	0 R	0 L	1 R	1 L	1+ R	1+ L	2 R	2 L	2+ R	2+ L	3 R	3 L	3+ R	3+ L	4 R	4 L	4+ R	4+ L	5 R	5 L
C4	Deltoid																				
C5	Biceps																				
C6	Ext. Carp Rad Long																				
C6	Pro. Teres																				
C7	Triceps																				
C7	Ext. Ind. Prop																				
C8	Flex Carp Uln																				
C8	Flex Dig Subl																				
T1	Opponens Pollicis																				
T1	Abd Dig V																				
T8–T10	Upper Abdom																				
T10–T12	Lower Abdom																				
L2	Iliopsoas																				
L3	Quadriceps																				
L4	Ant Tibialis																				
L5	Ext. Hall Long																				
S1	Gastroc																				

5 = normal   2 = full range gravity eliminated

4 = withstands some resistance   1 = palpable contraction

3 = full range antigravity   0 = no contraction

ANATOMICAL LEVEL OF FUNCTION:
(list the lowest, most caudal segment *above* the level of injury in which motor *and* sensory function are *normal*)

SENSORY LEVEL: _____

SACRAL SPARING: ____ YES ____ NO

NORMAL (PRESERVED) THROUGH:

ABLE TO VOID?   ____ YES ____ NO

     RIGHT   LEFT

RECTAL TONE?   ____ YES ____ NO

Table 3.1—*continued*

				COMMENTS

Sensory Level: _____   Sacral Sparing: _____ Yes _____ No

Able to Void? _____ Yes _____ No   Rectal Tone? _____ Yes _____ No

Reflex Withdrawal? _____ Yes _____ No

	Normal	Partial	Absent
Pin:	_____	_____	_____
Prop and/or Truck	_____	_____	_____

Reflexes:	Right	Left
Biceps	_____	_____
ECRL	_____	_____
Finger flex	_____	_____
Knee	_____	_____
Ankle	_____	_____

Plantar reflex	Up	Down	Absent
Right	_____	_____	_____
Left	_____	_____	_____

	Hyper	Normal	Hypo	Absent
Bulbocavernous	_____	_____	_____	_____
Anal wink	_____	_____	_____	_____

Spasticity: _____ Yes Interferes with _ Mobility _ Positioning
_____ No   _ ADL _ SOC

Spasticity:
With/clonus _____ Yes Interferes with _ Mobility _ Positioning
_ ADL _ SOC

Lesion type:
_ Upper motor neuron _ Lower motor neuron _ Undefined

Frankel grade (preserved neurological function):
_____ 0 = Not applicable (complete lesion)
_____ 1 = Preserved sensation only
_____ 2 = Preserved motor (nonfunctional)
_____ 3 = Preserved motor (functional)
_____ 4 = Complete neurological recovery
_____ 5 = Unknown

ASIA American Spinal Injury Association Motor Index Score	Grade on right	Muscle	Grade on left
	5	C5	5
	5	C6	5
	5	C7	5
	5	C8	5
	5	T1	5
	5	L2	5
	5	L3	5
	5	L4	5
	5	L5	5
	5	S1	5
	50		50

Clinical classification:

	Right	Left
Sensory level	_____	_____
Motor level	_____	_____
Motor index score	_____	_____
Total motor index score	_____	_____

If complete, zone of injury findings _____
If incomplete,
Functional classification _____
Anatomical Classification _____
(cord syndrome)

Anatomical level of function (list lowest, most caudal segment above the level of injury in which motor and sensory functions are normal ... i.e., > 3/5 MMT)
Right _____   Left _____
Signature _____ Date _____

mination of the level of motor and sensory function preserved and whether there is preservation below the level of injury. The "Standards for Neurological Classification of Spinal Injury Patients" developed by the American Spinal Injury Association in 1983 are recommended for use as a guideline and to ensure accurate and consistent communication regarding the patient's neurologic status. The standards recommend that the level of injury be defined as the "lowest (most caudal) neurological segment with both normal motor and sensory function." It should be noted that, for the purpose of this examination, a muscle grade of 3/5 or better is considered normal.

Determination of whether the patient's neurologic injury is *complete* or *incomplete* is important in dictating the optimal course of medical and surgical management in the acute phase of care. Utilization of the *Frankel Grading* system of functional classification is helpful in further understanding the patient's incomplete neurological status (Table 1.1), and the *Motor Index Score* provides even further descriptive information (Table 3.2).

The sensory examination should be based on the Austin illustration of dermatomal segmentation as recommended by the ASIA guidelines (see illustration). The presence or absence of sensory function in the perineal area should be ascertained to determine whether there is "sacral sparing" that is indicative of an incomplete spinal cord injury.

All deep-tendon and superficial reflexes, including the superficial abdominal, the cremasteric, the Babinski, and the bulbocavernosus reflex, should be carefully assessed. In the patient with SCI, the bulbocavernosus reflex may be elicited by gently tugging on the Foley catheter.

After the neurologic level and extent of injury have been carefully evaluated and documented, the orthopedic assessment of the injuries of the vertebral column and supporting structures should be initiated. If cervical spine injury is suspected, the initial radiographic evaluation should be done by performing a portable cross-table lateral x-ray of the cervical spine. The immobilization should not be removed, and

Table 3.2
Motor Index Score[a]

Grade on Right	Muscle	Grade on Left
5	C5—Biceps	5
5	C6—Ext. Carpi. Radialis	5
5	C7—Triceps	5
5	C8—Ext. Ind. Prop.	5
5	T1—Opponens Pollicis	5
5	L2—Iliopsoas	5
5	L3—Quadriceps	5
5	L4—Ant. Tibialis	5
5	L5—Ext. Hallicus Longus	5
5	S1—Gastrocnemius	5
50		50

Total Score = 100

[a] From "Standards for Neurological Classification of Spinal Injury Patients," Birmingham, AL, American Spinal Injury Association, October, 1982.

the patient should not be moved from the spinal board until this has been completed.

Adequate views of the first two vertebral bodies and the junction of the seventh cervical and first thoracic vertebral junction are imperative for a full evaluation. Conventional radiographic technology may be used, or some cases may require the more sophisticated use of tomography.

Persons suspected of having spinal injury below the cervical spine level may need to be moved to the x-ray suite in order to obtain adequate films. They may be screened with lateral thoracic and lumbar films and with anteroposterior views of the pelvis and chest. Linear tomography and/or computed tomography may be necessary to visualize the vertebral injuries fully.

Patients should be accompanied by experienced SCI personnel at all times during the assessment process. This is particularly important during the radiographic evaluation process. Remember, radiology technicians are trained to obtain optimal radiographs, but may not be equally skilled in ensuring that spinal alignment is maintained. It is preferred that an orthopedic physican or house staff member remain with the patient during the x-ray evaluation to supervise all patient movement, to ensure the acquisition of appropriate radiographic views, to monitor the patient's neurologic status, and to ensure patient safety.

A complete evaluation of the patient's pulmonary status is imperative to determine the degree of respiratory involvement secondary to the spinal cord injury. Because of involvement of the phrenic nerve, complete spinal cord injury at the first, second, or third cervical levels renders the person unable to breathe at all without ventilatory assistance. Injury to the cord at the fourth and fifth cervical levels also compromises the function of the phrenic nerve.

In cervical lesions, abdominal (paradoxical) breathing should be noted on examination. Full respiratory parameters should be measured as soon as possible. Of particular importance are arterial blood gas analysis and measurement of the vital capacity. Although the analysis of adequate vital capacity is dependent upon the patient's height and mass, as a rule of thumb, any vital capacity measurement of less than 1 liter should alert the clinician to repiratory difficulty and the possibility of impending ventilatory failure. Appropriate ventilatory support equipment, including a tracheostomy tray and mechanical ventilator, should be prepared, and appropriate respiratory medical personnel and a respiratory therapist should be available.

All patients should be evaluated for associated injuries of the chest that could cause impairment of respiratory function independently of the neurologic injury. Multiple rib fractures also may be accompanied by traumatic pneumothorax and/or hemopneumothorax. Patients with injuries of the thoracic spine are particularly susceptible to associated respiratory compromise and traumatic aortic aneurysm because of trauma to the chest.

Cardiovascular compromise should be carefully assessed in the ED. Hypotension secondary to spinal shock is usually accompanied by profound bradycardia. The adequacy of end-organ perfusion and mentation should be carefully evaluated to determine whether cardiac output is being severely compromised by the effects of the neurogenic shock. If end-organ perfusion and mentation are not compromised, the hypotension and bradycardic reaction should not be treated with the infusion of high volumes of i.v. fluids.

Associated injuries to the heart and great vessels of the neck and chest should be carefully assessed in cases of obvious chest trauma and when the force of impact at the time of injury was reportedly severe. Aortic aneurysm should be ruled out in cases of severe chest trauma.

Continuous cardiac monitoring is important for all patients with acute spinal cord injury. Some patients with traumatic spinal cord injury may need the assistance of a temporary cardiac pacemaker to prevent episodes of life-threatening bradycardia. Vasopressor medications are rarely necessary to maintain an adequate blood pressure in the case of neurogenic shock, but the possibility should not be overlooked.

Gastrointestinal ileus occurs in many SCI patients. Onset is usually immediate, and the ileus may persist for several days to a week postinjury. The presence or absence of bowel sounds should be carefully assessed during the ED evaluation.

The potential for gastrointestinal bleeding in persons with traumatic spinal cord injury must be addressed in the emergency phase of care. Historically, the incidence of gastrointestinal bleeding is extremely high, with a significant percentage of persons with spinal cord injury requiring surgical intervention for the treatment of gastric stress ulcers. It has been demonstrated that the early initiation of prophylaxis significantly reduces the incidence of gastrointestinal bleeding. Cimetidine 300 mg intravenously, given during the emergency phase of care and continued throughout the acute care phase, serves this purpose in the majority of cases.

Genitourinary compromise is an immediate effect of acute spinal cord injury. At the time of injury, the bladder is rendered atonic, and the patient experiences either urinary incontinence or retention. An indwelling Foley catheter should be inserted as soon after injury as possible to prevent overdistension of the bladder. The catheter should be connected to straight drainage with a system setup that allows for careful monitoring of urinary output.

The possibility of trauma to the kidneys, ureters, and bladder should be carefully assessed in obvious or suspected cases of blunt trauma to the abdomen. A complete urinalysis should be obtained in the ED, and the urine should be tested for the presence of blood. A more complete urologic evaluation can be ordered once significant trauma has been ruled out.

Male patients with acute spinal cord injury often experience immediate priapism. Although the patient may believe that this is a sign of positive potential sexual function, priapism in the initial phase following injury is usually associated with complete spinal cord injury. If the injury occurs in the sacral segment of the spinal cord, the patient may present with flaccidity of the penis. A more comprehensive evaluation of sexual function can be carried out later in the patient's hospital stay. In the emergency phase of care, however, trauma to the genitalia must be assessed and treated.

A full evaluation for the presence of associated injuries of the head, chest, abdomen, and extremities should be done in the ED. It is important to remember that the insensate patient cannot report or describe the pain of injury below the level of the injured spinal cord.

The possibility of concomitant head injury should be ruled out by an experienced neurologic surgeon. In the case of reported or obvious head trauma, a CT scan of the head may be required in the emergency phase of care to determine whether immediate intervention is necessary. Some authorities believe that the incidence of occult brain trauma in persons with spinal cord trauma is much higher than previously believed. Cognitive deficits have been identified late in the rehabilitation process in some persons with no identified head injury at the time of injury.

Extremity fractures should be thoroughly assessed and treated by an experienced orthopedic surgeon. Because the person with paralysis may become primarily dependent on his or her upper extremities for moving the body mass, even small fractures of the hands and wrists can assume enormous significance if they are not appropriately identified and addressed in the emergency phase of care.

It is important to obtain an accurate and complete medical history of the patient. If the injured person cannot cooperate, the patient's family or friends should be interviewed. A history of major system compromise, such as cardiovascular, pulmonary, renal, or neuromusculoskeletal disease, significantly affects the patient's initial assessment and care in the emergency phase, as well as throughout the hospitalization.

A significant history of psychiatric disorder and drug and/or alcohol use and abuse is important. The neurologic assessment of mental status may be unreliable based on consumption of alcohol or medications before the injury. Patients who are severely intoxicated or who are less than fully alert because of the use of medications cannot adequately participate in the neurologic examination. In such cases the initial neurologic evaluation must be considered suspect.

Safety precautions must be initiated for patients with a significant history of psychiatric problems and/or drug and alcohol abuse. For example, the person who has a history of alcohol abuse or heroin use may require medication to prevent severe withdrawal symptoms.

Regardless of whether there are associated injuries, traumatic spinal cord injury affects every major system of the body. It is extremely important that a thorough clinical, radiographic, and laboratory assessment of the patient's status be completed as soon after injury as possible. Because spinal cord injury is a multisystem problem, appropriate treatment requires a multidisciplinary and multispecialty management approach.

After completing the assessment, attention should be directed toward the immobilization and stabilization of the patient's injuries.

Medical stabilization is, of course, of paramount importance. As previously mentioned, the cardiovascular, pulmonary, gastrointestinal, and genitourinary effects of the spinal cord injury and associated injuries should be addressed first.

STABILIZATION

Stabilization of the neurologic injury can be accomplished simultaneously with immobilization. The following procedures may be instituted in the ED: (a) insertion of an indwelling Foley catheter, (b) starting an i.v. line with a solution of 5% dextrose and .2 normal saline to run via minidropper at a rate of 30 minidrops/min, (c) administration of Decadron 10 mg i.v., (d) administration of 1 ampule of sodium bicarbonate (NaHCO3) i.v., (e) administration of Mannitol 50 g i.v. if the systolic blood pressure is greater than 110 mm Hg, (f) insertion of a nasogastric tube if the patient is to be transferred to another hospital or SCI Center and (g) provision of oxygen via mask or cannula if the blood oxygen saturation level is substandard.

It is important to communicate with the patient's family and/or significant others during the emergency phase of care. Often, the family may have no idea of the severity of the injury when the patient is taken to the hospital. It is not only kind but it is also important to secure the family's trust, support, and cooperation by meeting with them as soon as possible to discuss the results of the initial assessment and the immediate plan of care. The physician should meet with the family in the ED. A more comprehensive family meeting can be arranged after the patient has been formally admitted to the hospital.

TRANSPORT

Transport is the final step of the emergency phase of care, regardless of whether the patient is being transferred to an intensive care unit within the same hospital or to another facility. It is important that the patient be appropriately immobilized and monitored during the transport process. Whenever possible, a physician or critical care nurse should accompany the patient during all transport activities.

If the patient is to be referred to another hospital or SCI Center, it is recommended that the referring physician *not* institute cervical traction before transfer. The patient can be most safely transported in the emergency phase of care by being firmly secured to a long spinal board with a collar and sandbags to maintain spinal alignment. A high level of experience and expertise—and the appropriate equipment—is required to transfer a patient with an unstable spine in cervical traction.

If the patient is to be transferred to another hospital or SCI Center, it is important to call the receiving facility as soon as possible after the patient arrives in the ED. The receiving personnel will review the recommended guidelines for preadmission care and will work with the referring facility to coordinate the transfer process. Some SCI Centers have an emergency retrieval team that goes to the referring facility to pick up the acutely injured patient.

It is helpful to acquire the SCI Center's emergency referral guidelines and develop an organizational policy regarding the triage of acute SCI patients before a patient arrives. Doing so minimizes confusion and allows for optimal availability of patient transfer resources.

Management in the Critical Care Environment

In the critical care environment, comprehensive evaluation and treatment should be directed toward medical, neurologic, and orthopedic stabilization and the prevention of the life-threatening and long-term debilitating complications of traumatic spinal cord injury. The stabilization efforts that were begun in the emergency phase should continue and be expanded in the acute phase of care. It is important to remember that ongoing assessment is imperative in the acute care phase regarding all three aspects of stabilization. Two to 7 days may be required before a person with acute spinal cord injury may truly be considered stable.

MEDICAL STABILIZATION

Continuous monitoring of the patient's cardiovascular status is imperative. The staff should carefully assess the patient for the effects of hypotension, bradycardia, and decreased cardiac output. Appropriate resuscitation equipment, including equipment for the emergency insertion of a temporary cardiac pacemaker, should be available and ready for use at all times.

The ongoing assessment of the respiratory status of the acutely injured person with confirmed or suspected cervical injury should include a baseline arterial blood gas analysis and serial monitoring of the respiratory parameters every 4 hr around the clock for at least the first 48 to 72 hr. Persons with cervical injuries who do not require mechanical ventilation at admission may experience fatigue of the diaphragm within the first 72 hr and may require ventilatory support subsequently. Careful serial monitoring of the respiratory parameters can alert the staff to the impending crisis and allow appropriate intervention to be instituted to prevent the need for emergency response.

Patients with a history of pulmonary disease or those with severe abdominal distention that may compromise diaphragmatic function should be carefully monitored. The presence of these risk factors should be noted at the time of admission.

NEUROLOGIC STABILIZATION

It is important that the patient's neurologic status be monitored on an hourly basis for the first 24 hr and then every 4 hr for the next 48 hr. Neurologic findings may fluctuate in extent and/or level, or they may remain constant. Any change in neurologic status should be noted and reported to the physician immediately. Persons with symptoms of deteriorating neurologic function may require immediate surgical intervention.

Figure 3.1 is an example of an assessment tool that can be utilized by the nursing staff in the critical care environment for documenting the ongoing assessment of the patient's neurologic status. The format of the nursing assessment is similar to that recommended in Chapter 2 for paramedical personnel. It is based upon an assessment of function, rather than the grading of the strength of specific muscles. It is important that, if such a tool is utilized, the first examination of the patient be performed with the patient's physician in order to ensure accuracy in communication.

Steroid and diuretic therapy may be continued for at least the first 72 hr after injury in order to reduce the existing edema of the spinal cord and to minimize the risk of further neurologic deficit as a result of spinal cord edema. Intravenous fluids should be minimized for the same reason. After 72 hr, the steroid and diuretic medication may be discontinued if the patient's lesion has been confirmed to be complete.

The indications for neurologic spinal surgery at the time of admission are (a) deteriorating neurologic function and (b) evidence of bone, disk, or other matter in the neural canal with compression of the spinal cord in the presence of an incomplete injury. The person with a complete spinal cord injury may require neurosurgical intervention at the time of surgical fusion to restore the integrity of the neural canal and to prevent long-term problems with spinal pain and deformity.

ORTHOPEDIC STABILIZATION

Definitive orthopedic reduction and/or stabilization efforts may not be initiated until the patient arrives in the ICU when the initial immobilization devices may be removed safely. If fracture or fracture dislocation reduction is necessary, it is often best to perform it within the intensive care environment. Doing so allows for the availability of appropriate support staff and equipment in a controlled environment, rather than in the often chaotic atmosphere of the ED.

Cervical spine reduction efforts may be monitored utilizing portable x-ray equipment. Gardner-Wells tongs may be inserted in the ICU. Often the reduction is performed after transferring the patient to the appropriate bed for optimal immobilization and management of the patient (STRYKER turning frame, ROTO-REST bed, etc.). Spinal reduction is often a time-consuming process as additional weights are added to the cervical traction and serial x-rays are evaluated. Careful clinical and radiographic monitoring during the reduction process are essential.

In some cases, surgery is necessary to reduce a fracture-dislocation that does not respond adequately to closed reduction efforts. If indicated, definitive internal fixation of the vertebral column with decompression of the spinal canal may be postponed until the patient is medically stable and can best withstand the risk of the surgical procedure.

Once adequate spinal reduction has been achieved, a turning schedule for the patient must be established. The risk of pressure sore development should not be overlooked in the acute phase of care.

REGIONAL SPINAL CORD INJURY CENTER

NURSING NEURO WATCH FLOW SHEET

ADDRESSOGRAPH

FUNCTION	MUSCLE	LEVEL	DATE:												
			TIME:												
			L/R	L/R	L/R	L/R	L/R	L/R	L/R	L/R	L/R	L/R	L/R	L/R	L/R
Shoulder Shrug	Trapezius Levator Scap.	CN X1 C3–4													
Raise Arms	Deltoids	C4													
Elbow Flexion	Biceps	C5													
Wrist Dorsiflexion	Ext. Carpi Rad. Long	C6													
Elbow Extension	Triceps	C7													
Thumb-Index Pinch	Opponens Poll. Flex. Dig. Subl.	C8–T1													
Upper Abdominals	Rectus Abdominus	T8–T10													
Lower Abdominals	Rectus Abdominus	T10–T12													
Hip Flexion	Iliopsoas	L2													
Knee Extension	Quadriceps	L3													
Ankle Dorsiflexion	Ant. Tibialis	L4													
Knee Flexion	Hamstrings	L5, S1													
Ankle Dorsiflexion	Gastroc.	S1													

Anocutaneous	Pudendal (Sensory)	S2–4
Bulbocaver-nosus	Pudendal (Motor)	S2–4
Other		
Fasciculation		
Tone		
Atrophy		

5 = Normal—Complete ROM against gravity with full resistance
4 = Good—Complete ROM against gravity with some resistance
3 = Fair—Complete ROM against gravity
2 = Poor—Complete ROM with gravity eliminated
1 = Trace—Evidence of contraction. No joint movement.
0 = Zero—No evidence of contraction

Figure 3.1. Nursing neuro watch.

Alternative beds, such as the STRYKER turning frame and the ROTO-REST bed, may facilitate the turning of the patient, but care must be taken not to assume that technology can replace the hands-on care necessary to prevent pressure sores. Skin care must be initiated from the onset of acute care in order to prevent costly, debilitating, and life-threatening pressure sores.

Alternative Beds.   The person with traumatic spinal cord injury may be immobilized initially in the ICU on a regular hospital bed or on an alternative bed designed to provide for safe turning and patient care. There are several alternative beds currently in use. Each has its own indications, advantages, and disadvantages.

The STRYKER turning frame is a two-piece metal frame covered with canvas (Fig. 3.2). The anterior and posterior frames can be bolted and strapped together with the patient "sandwiched" in between. The STRYKER frame allows the patient to be turned laterally from the supine to prone position by two staff members for pressure relief and skin care. The patient can be immobilized in cervical and extremity traction on the STRYKER frame.

It has been shown that a person may experience a 25% reduction in pulmonary vital capacity when turned to the prone position. For this reason, use of the STRYKER frame in persons with marginal vital capacity and/or cardiovascular instability is ill advised. It is also difficult for the average person to exercise full range of shoulder joint motion while immobilized on the STRYKER frame because of the presence of the metal frame. The recommended weight limit for the STRYKER frame is 250 pounds. A person with greater than average body mass must be carefully assessed to ensure that pressure sores at the shoulders are not developing.

The CIRCO-ELECTRIC bed is a motorized frame with anterior and posterior halves that turn the patient vertically from the supine to the prone position. The use of the "circle" bed is not recommended for the management of persons with spinal cord injury because of the axial loading effect on the spine during the turning process. For the patient

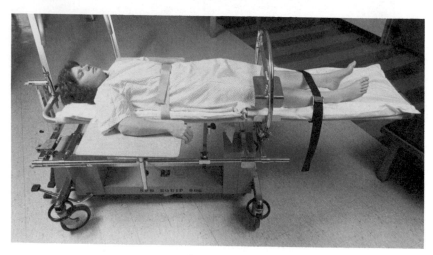

Figure 3.2.   STRYKER turning frame.

immobilized in cervical traction, it is difficult to control the weights safely during the turn.

The ROTO-REST bed (KINETIC TREATMENT TABLE) is a motorized turning bed that rotates the patient through an arc of 140–160° every 3 to 4 min (Fig. 3.3). It is important to understand that the bed must be in motion a minimum of 20 hr out of each 24-hr period in order to achieve the appropriate treatment effects for the prevention of pressure sores. The patient is secured in place by vinyl bolsters that are inserted into the surface of the bed. Care must be taken to secure the patient firmly in position on the bed to prevent the deleterious shearing effect that may cause skin breakdown.

Immobilization with cervical and extremity traction can be more easily maintained on the ROTO-REST without the risk of respiratory compromise that may occur when the patient is turned to the prone position. In fact, use of the ROTO-REST bed may improve respiratory function by assisting in the mobilization of pulmonary secretions. It has been noted that a marked mobilization of secretions occurs in the first few hours after the patient is placed on the ROTO-REST bed.

However, patients immobilized on the ROTO-REST bed may develop symptoms of motion sickness that can be treated with such medication as Dramamine. Overstimulation effects, such as mental confusion and sleeplessness, may contribute to the disorienting effects of the continuous motion of the bed and the intensive care environment. If this occurs, it may be necessary to remove the patient from the ROTO-REST bed and the environment, if possible.

The alternative beds described above are recommended for short-term use. Because of the difficulty in mobilizing the patient and in encouraging independence in self-care and transfer activities while in these beds, the patient should be transferred to a standard adjustable hospital bed when stability of the spine has been achieved.

Spinal Orthoses. Application of a definitive spinal orthosis may

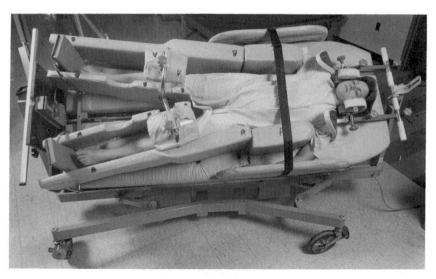

Figure 3.3. ROTO-REST bed (kinetic treatment table).

precede, follow, or eliminate the need for surgical stabilization. Commonly used orthoses include the halo vest, the SOMI, the Philadelphia collar, and a custom-fitted plastic body jacket.

The halo vest is a self-contained traction device that allows the unstable spine to be immobilized rigidly while permitting the patient to be mobilized (Fig. 3.4). The halo is a stainless steel ring that is secured to the outer table of the skull with four surgical steel screws. Vertical steel struts connect the halo ring to a plastic body jacket that is lined with sheepskin. Once the halo vest has been applied and stabilization of the spine has been radiographically confirmed, the patient may be managed on a regular hospital bed. Mobilization to a sitting position and out of bed in a chair is permitted once the orthopedic surgeon determines that the patient's spine is stable in the halo brace.

The SOMI (sterno-occipital-mandibular-immobilizer) brace is utilized when immobilization is needed (Fig. 3.5). Often, the SOMI is used to limit flexion and extension when control of rotation is less of a concern. Constructed of plastic occipital and mandibular supports and steel struts that connect the supports to a plate that rests on the chest, the SOMI allows for early mobilization.

The Philadelphia collar and similar collars may be the only immobilization needed preoperatively if there is not severe spinal instability, or it may be needed postoperatively when internal fixation has been accomplished (Fig. 3.6). Constructed of anterior and posterior plastic halves that are secured wtih Velcro straps, the Philadelphia collar prohibits gross flexion, extension, and rotation when it is properly fitted and applied.

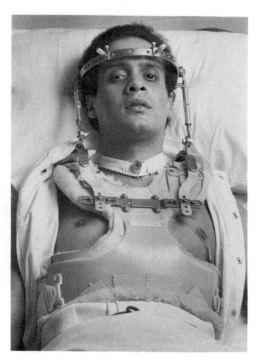

Figure 3.4. Halo-vest.

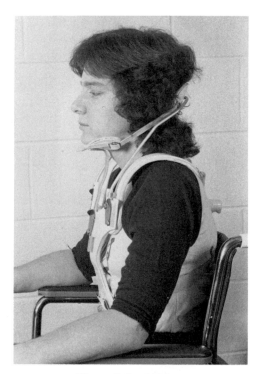

Figure 3.5. SOMI.

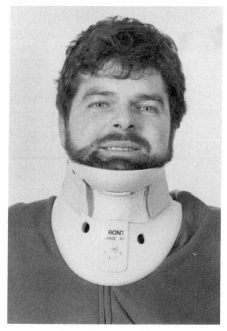

Figure 3.6. Philadelphia collar.

A custom-fitted plastic body jacket is indicated in patients with injuries to the vertebral column below the cervical and upper thoracic levels (Fig. 3.7). Bi-valved and secured with Velcro straps, the plastic body jacket (or "turtle shell" or "clam shell") can be opened to allow

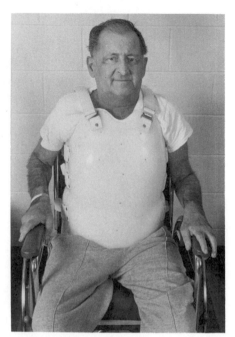

Figure 3.7.   Custom-made body jacket.

for washing and skin inspection. It is recommended for use with insensate persons who are at risk of developing skin breakdown. Traditionally, plaster body casts had been used that did not allow for skin inspection and cleaning.

Immobilization with a spinal orthosis is required until the patient's vertebral injuries heal and the neural elements of the spinal cord are no longer at risk of further damage. Most patients require 8–16 weeks for stability to be achieved. It is important that the orthopedic surgeon evaluate the stability of the patient's spine at regular intervals to determine when it is safe to remove the orthosis.

Prevention Of Complications In The Acute Phase

Major complications of spinal cord injury affect nearly every body system and must begin to be addressed by the multidisciplinary team during the acute phase of care. In order to minimize the risks of morbidity, mortality, and the debilitating compromise of maximal health and function, appropriate prophylaxis, early assessment, and therapeutic intervention are essential.

Some complications result from the injury to the spinal cord, whereas others are a consequence of the immobilization that is required during the initial phase of care. Still others are the result of a combination of these factors.

RESPIRATORY COMPLICATIONS

Respiratory complications are the primary cause of death acutely in persons with traumatic spinal cord injury. Aggressive assessment and prevention efforts are required to minimize the risk of respiratory death.

Patients with lesions of the spinal cord at the first, second, or third cervical levels are unable to breathe without the assistance of a mechanical ventilator because of injury at or above the level of the phrenic nerve. Those with injuries above T1 have lost or diminished innervation to the intercostal muscles of respiration and may require short-term mechanical ventilation assistance because of fatigue of the diaphragm. All persons with quadriplegia with or without ventilator-dependence and those with high-level paraplegia who require rigid stabilization of the thorax are at great risk of pulmonary infection and respiratory death.

Atelectasis, pneumonia, and *ventilatory failure* may occur because of the patient's inability to cough effectively, decreased movement of the diaphragm, and diminished vital capacity. A positive history of pulmonary disease, smoking, and/or aspiration may contribute to respiratory problems.

Prevention is key. Aggressive respiratory assessment and pulmonary care directed toward minimizing the retention of pulmonary secretions are imperative to compensate for the loss of functional intercostal and abdominal musculature. With attentive monitoring of pulmonary parameters and aggressive pulmonary management, the effects of respiratory complications can be minimized or prevented entirely. (See Chapter 5 for prevention and intervention strategies.)

Respiratory management should also include the assessment of the need for elective tracheotomy. If it is anticipated that mechanical ventilation or endotracheal or nasotracheal intubation will be required for longer than 10 days, a tracheotomy may need to be performed to prevent the long-term complication of *tracheal stenosis*. The need for prolonged medical and surgical intervention can be avoided by preventing erosion of the tracheal wall in the acute phase of care.

CARDIOVASCULAR COMPLICATIONS

Bradycardia and *hypotension* are features of neurogenic shock that result from the disruption of sympathetic innervation. With peripheral vasodilation, venous pooling, and decreased cardiac output, both the heart rate and blood pressure are significantly reduced. In persons with spinal cord injury below the level of T6, bradycardia and hypotension are not usually significant, although cardiovascular assessment is necessary.

Some persons with lesions of the cervical cord may exhibit a vasovagal response leading to profound bradycardia and cardiac arrest with a abrupt position change, prone positioning, and suctioning. It is believed that cardiac changes are caused by the loss of sympathetic innervation and the resultant parasympathetic override. As previously stated, continuous cardiac monitoring is imperative in the first 24–72 hr after traumatic spinal cord injury. A full assessment of cardiac function is recommended.

Deep-vein thrombosis (DVT) is a major cardiovascular complication of spinal cord injury. It occurs when the venous system of the lower extremities is occluded by clot formation. Major contributing factors are decreased or absent muscle function in the legs and loss of sympathetic innervation after spinal cord injury that leads to vasodilation and pooling of blood in the venous system. Hypercoagulability and trauma may also be contributing factors.

Estimates of the incidence of DVT range from 40% to nearly 100% of SCI patients. Recent studies indicate that the person with motor complete quadriplegia has the greatest likelihood of developing DVT. Undetected and untreated DVT may lead to pulmonary embolus and sudden death. Early identification can ensure that the appropriate therapeutic intervention is initiated.

The clinical signs of DVT, such as thigh or calf swelling, elevated temperature, and localized warmth of the extremity, are diagnostic in only about 15% of cases. Attentive screening may include serial I-125 fibrinogen scans and impedance plethysmography (IPG), as well as the careful documentation of clinical symptoms. Positive findings by screening studies suggestive of DVT should be confirmed by venography.

At this time there is little evidence that prophylactic low-dose heparin, antiembolic stockings, and passive range of motion to the lower extremities significantly reduce the incidence or severity of DVT. Therefore, early diagnosis is recommended for the prompt initiation of therapeutic levels of anticoagulation. In those patients for whom anticoagulation is contraindicated, the insertion of a Greenfield filter into the inferior vena cava may be necessary to prevent pulmonary emboli.

GASTROINTESTINAL COMPLICATIONS

Gastrointestinal (GI) *bleeding* is a preventable complication of traumatic spinal cord injury. Before the development of cimetidine, the formation of stress ulcers was a frequent complication. Treatment required the infusion of antacids and strict dietary control. Surgical repair or subtotal gastrectomy was often required. At this time, however, the incidence of GI bleeding has been reduced to less than 5% in patients who receive cimetidine prophylactically.

Although the specific cause of stress ulcers has not been proven, it has been postulated that steroid therapy, emotional stress, loss of sympathetic innervation to the GI tract, and mechanical ventilation are primary contributing factors. Patients with a history of ulcer disease are more prone to bleeding problems. Anticoagulation also increases the risk of GI bleeding. It is important that all patients be carefully screened by testing for occult blood in stool and stomach contents and by carefully monitoring their hemoglobin and hematocrit levels.

The GI tract is frequently rendered atonic at the time of injury. *Ileus* may accompany neurogenic shock. Marked by the absence of bowel sounds for the first 24 to 72 hr, the ileus may persist and require gastric decompression. Careful assessment of the GI tract is necessary to determine the appropriate timing for the initiation of a bowel program and to prevent constipation and/or obstruction. The bowel program should be started as soon as bowel sounds return and the patient is receiving oral feedings.

Nutritional considerations must be addressed from the onset of acute care. It is important to ensure optimal healing responses and to prevent the long-term complications of inadequate nutrition. Nasogastric feedings or total parenteral nutrition (TPN) via a central venous line may be necessary if the patient cannot tolerate oral intake by the fifth day after injury.

GENITOURINARY COMPLICATIONS

The flaccid paralysis of the urinary bladder that occurs at the time of traumatic spinal cord injury persists in persons with upper motor neuron lesions until the phase of neurogenic (spinal) shock resolves. After the initial phase of flaccidity, the bladder becomes spastic. In the case of a lower motor neuron lesion, the bladder remains atonic.

During the acute phase of care, it is important that bladder function be carefully assessed and treatment initiated to prevent life-threatening and long-term complications of the genitourinary tract. Bladder infection can progress to pyelonephritis, septicemia, and death in the acute phase or may become a chronic problem, presenting a continuing threat to the patient's life and well-being.

While the patient is receiving steroid, diuretic, and i.v. therapy, urinary output must be carefully monitored. Overdistention of the bladder must be avoided, and fluid balance must be achieved. The Foley catheter that is inserted in the emergency phase should remain in place until medical and neurologic stabilization are achieved. The closed system of the catheter and drainage setup should be maintained and changed every 3 days to avoid infection of the urine.

It has been shown that an indwelling catheter causes localized infection in the bladder after a period of 48 to 72 hr. Prolonged use of an indwelling catheter may result in contracture and atrophy of the bladder musculature. For these reasons, the indwelling catheter should be discontinued as soon as it is deemed appropriate in regard to the patient's overall medical/surgical management.

As soon as the phase of diuresis is over, the catheter should be removed, and a program of bladder retraining with intermittent catheterization and fluid restriction should be initiated. A complete urologic evaluation should be performed before the start of bladder retraining. Scrupulous attention to the prevention of bladder infection and overdistention is essential. Urinary tract infections should be identified and treated with appropriate therapy.

MUSCULOSKELETAL AND INTEGUMENTARY COMPLICATIONS

Pressure sores and *joint contractures* are often the most debilitating and costly complications of traumatic spinal cord injury. They are also preventable with appropriate prophylactic intervention beginning in the acute phase of care.

It has been estimated that a single pressure sore can cost as much as $30,000 if surgical repair is necessary. The onset of physical rehabilitation may be delayed by the need for prolonged bedrest, the initial hospitalization may be extended, and the psychological adjustment process may be more complicated than necessary.

Pressure sore prevention is often considered to be a primary responsibility of the nursing staff. Without question, nurses must assume responsibility for planning and implementing appropriate turning, hygiene, and skin care activities. However, it is imperative that the entire multidisciplinary team ensure that the integrity of the patient's skin is not compromised.

Pressure sores can develop as early as the emergency phase of care if definitive diagnosis and treatment are delayed. Adequate stabilization must be achieved as soon as possible after injury to ensure that the patient can be safely turned. Alternative beds should be prescribed to facilitate patient turning. The application of spinal orthoses should be carefully monitored to prevent the creation of pressure points.

Skin integrity should be assessed by every member of the treatment team to monitor the effects of the overall status of the management plan. The required immobilization, stabilization, and medical interventions may contribute to a loss of skin integrity. The nutritional and metabolic status of the patient may be reflected in the status of the skin. For these reasons, skin integrity must be a concern of every member of the team.

Joint contractures are also fully preventable with appropriate early prophylaxis. Proper positioning, the use of such immobilization aids as foam booties and positioning pillows, and range of motion exercises can prevent the contracture of peripheral joints. Aggressive range of motion of the shoulders and hips should be instituted as soon as it is determined that it will not present a risk to the unstable vertebral column.

Loss of joint motion can result in deformity below the level of injury and can seriously impair mobilization efforts. Contractures above the level of injury can impair the patient's functional capabilities.

PSYCHOSOCIAL COMPLICATIONS

The psychosocial complications of traumatic spinal cord injury affect and are affected by every aspect of the patient's management, as well as by his or her premorbid life experiences. Denial, depression, and anger may be manifested in ways that compromise the management plan and overall well-being of the patient. Consideration of the psychosocial reaction and adjustment process to the injury must not be delayed.

Every effort should be made to involve the patient and family in the development of the management plan whenever possible. Many patients are anxious to be informed about their conditions and the required treatment program. Others are unable to cope with this information in the initial phase of care. Careful assessment and recognition of the patient's emotional status are imperative.

Family members and significant others must be informed of the patient's diagnosis and prognosis as soon as possible in order to enlist their understanding, support, and cooperation. If the family is appropriately informed and supported, the medical/surgical and rehabilitation management plan can be developed with a better understanding of the patient.

It is important that all members of the treatment staff present a positive attitude to the patient. Attempts should be made to develop an atmosphere of trust and confidence. Predicted abilities should be stressed when discussing the injury and its effects, rather than emphasizing the obvious losses.

By addressing and considering the psychosocial impact of the injury on the patient early in the treatment program, the long-term adjustment to disability process is facilitated. Providing psychosocial support is the responsibility of every team member.

Team Approach to Comprehensive Care

The medical/surgical management of the person with traumatic spinal cord injury is a multispecialty, multidisciplinary team process. Each member of the physician team should provide the patient with high-level care within his or her area of expertise and should clearly understand that the scope of the multisystem problems requires the concerted expertise of a coordinated team.

In the acute phase of care, the roles of the neurologic and orthopedic surgeons are clearly definable. Working together, these physicians can best ensure optimal neurologic and orthopedic stabilization of the acutely injured person. Medical stabilization should be addressed by the primary physician in consultation with appropriate medical/surgical specialists.

Early intervention by rehabilitation medicine physicians working with the neurologic and orthopedic surgeons ensures that a comprehensive management approach is utilized and that the principles of rehabilitation are initiated. The status of the patient's neurologic level, immobilization, bladder and bowel function, lungs, and extremities should be assessed on a daily basis during the acute care phase by rehabilitation medicine physicians in order to assist the patient to achieve the highest possible level of health and fitness for the rehabilitation phase of care.

The rehabilitation medicine physician may assume primary responsibility for coordinating patient and family communication. Because the patient and family need to understand the long-term effects of the spinal cord injury and because most of the patient's hospitalization and follow-up care is provided by the rehabilitation team, it is important to establish trust and cooperation as early as possible.

During the emergency phase rehabilitation medicine physicians may best be involved in the patient's care by participating in the development of the overall management plan. A specific, individualized rehabilitation plan and prescription for the involvement of the rehabilitation allied health professionals are necessary at the time of admission. Intervention by occupational therapists, physical therapists, social workers, psychologists, and speech pathologists at the bedside should begin within the first 24 hr after injury in order to assist the newly injured person to achieve optimal functional and psychosocial outcomes. Working closely with the critical care nursing and medical/ surgical personnel, the rehabilitation team should serve to meet the patient's needs in a coordinated approach. A high level of communication and collaboration is essential.

At the same time that the acute medical/surgical issues of traumatic spinal cord injury are being addressed, every effort should be made to facilitate the patient's readiness for the ongoing rehabilitation process. The prevention of medical complications in the acute phase of care allows the person with traumatic spinal cord injury to participate fully in the rehabilitation program and to return to community living without unnecessary delay.

It has been demonstrated that coordination of team efforts from the onset of emergency care can result in a shortened hospitalization and rehabilitation period and can significantly decrease the costs of care for the injured individual, the family, and for society.

Suggested Readings

Carol M, Ducker TB, Byrnes DP: Acute care of spinal cord injury: A challenge to the emergency medicine clinician. *Crit Care Q* 2:7–21, June, 1979.

Ditunno JL: Spinal cord injury. In Ruskin AP (ed): *Current Therapy in Physiatry.* Philadelphia, WB Saunders, 1984.

Giubilato RT: Acute care of the high-level quadriplegic patient. *J Neurosurg Nurs* 14:128– 132, 1982.

Guttman Sir L: *Spinal Cord Injuries: Comprehensive Management and Research.* London, Blackwell Scientific Publications, 1973.

Pires M: Spinal cord injuries: Coping with devastating damage. In *Coping With Neurologic Problems Proficiently, Horsham,* Intermed Comm., 1980, p. 99.

Richmond TS: A critical care challenge: The patient with a cervical spinal cord injury. *Focus Crit Care,* 12:23–33, 1985.

Standards For Neurological Classification Of Spinal Injury Patient. Birmingham, AL, American Spinal Injury Association, 1983.

Stover SL: Spinal cord injury. *Cont Educ* 1:54–63, 1978.

Chapter 4

Respiratory Care

MARGARET E. RINEHART, M.S., P.T.
DEBORAH A. NAWOCZENSKI,
M.Ed., P.T.

Respiratory complications are a serious threat to the patient with spinal cord injury, and respiratory death is the leading cause of mortality. Each member of the health care team plays an integral role in the acute management phase of recovery for the patient who is adjusting to an altered respiratory system because of spinal cord injury.

When a spinal cord injury occurs at the high thoracic or cervical level, there may be paralysis of the intercostal muscles, abdominal muscles, and/or diaphragm that may lead to acute respiratory failure. If a patient survives the acute stage of respiratory distress, chronic problems may arise that may lead to complications of the respiratory system. These problems include the retention of secretions, atelectasis, and pneumonia. Therefore, many of the procedures incorporated into the early phase of management are frequently required throughout the individual's lifetime.

Promoting optimal respiratory function and preventing complications are the primary goals of the rehabilitation process. This chapter highlights the major intervention strategies in the respiratory treatment of the person with spinal cord injury.

Before assessing the respiratory status of the patient and establishing treatment goals, it is important that the clinician understands the muscles and normal mechanics of respiration. Knowledge of the level of the lesion provides an indication of which muscles may have impaired function, what compensations may occur, and the potential problems that can be anticipated.

Mechanics of Respiration

Respiration has two phases: *inspiration* and *expiration*. During normal breathing, inspiration is an active process involving the contraction of the major muscles, the *diaphragm* (innervated by the phrenic nerve, C3–5), and *external intercostals* (innervated by the intercostal nerves, T1–12).

Contraction of the diaphragm causes it to descend. As a result of this descent, the vertical diameter of the thoracic cavity increases, causing a decrease in the intrathoracic pressure. Air is then drawn into the lungs. At the same time, the abdominal contents are compressed, resulting in an increase in the intra-abdominal pressure.

The external intercostal muscles elevate the ribs during quiet inspiration. Their contraction causes an increase in the lateral and anteroposterior diameter of the thorax that creates a negative pressure gradient in the thoracic cavity. The negative pressure gradient also results in air flow into the lungs.

The diaphragm and external intercostals are the "active" muscles in normal inspiration. However, with a compromised respiratory system, the patient uses the accessory muscles of inspiration to assist with ventilation. These muscles act to elevate the ribs and include the *sternocleidomastoid*, the *scaleni*, and *trapezii*, the *pectoralis minor*, and the *serratus anterior*. The use of the accessory muscles in quiet inspiration is a clear indicator of impaired breathing.

Normally, expiration is a passive process unless active contraction of the respiratory muscles is needed to cough, sneeze, or expel secretions. The major muscles that contribute to expiration are the *abdominals* (T7–T11) and the *internal intercostals* (intercostal nerves T1–T12).

During forced expiration, the diaphragm is pushed up into the thoracic cavity by contraction of the abdominal muscles. The ribs are depressed by contraction of the internal intercostal muscles, resulting in a decrease in the lateral and anteroposterior diameter of the thorax.

Maintenance of good bronchial hygiene depends on the patient's ability to generate a strong, expiratory force and to maintain adequate chest wall mobility. A patient with a high thoracic or cervical cord injury may have significant compromise of these activities.

PATHOMECHANICS OF RESPIRATION

A patient with a high thoracic or low cervical spinal cord injury may have intercostal and abdominal muscle paralysis. The paralysis causes a decrease in both inspiratory and expiratory flow. Consequently, tidal volume and vital capacity measurements are reduced. Chest wall mobility may also be impaired because of intercostal muscle weakness or paralysis, and frequently, the patient cannot cough with enough force to clear secretions.

If there is abdominal muscle paralysis, changes in the patient's position affect the distribution of the visceral contents and the resting length of the diaphragm. In the supine position, the abdominal contents force the diaphragm to a higher resting level than in the upright or erect position. Therefore, there will be greater diaphragmatic excursion in the supine than in the upright position. The upright position creates a greater demand on the diaphragm as the downward pull of the abdominal contents by gravity causes the diaphragm to be in a lower resting position. Because of the lack of abdominal tone to support visceral contents, which in turn support the diaphragm, the diaphragm does not return to its normal resting position. Diaphragmatic excursion is decreased and is accompanied by a reduction in the patient's inspiratory capacity.

Adequate support must be provided for the viscera, and some mechanism needs to be adapted to substitute for the loss of abdominal tone so that ventilation is not severely compromised. Until the patient's respiratory capacity is strengthened, abdominal binders or corsets may be used to minimize the effects of gravity and provide support to the weak or absent abdominal muscles in the upright position.

Respiratory Assessment

An accurate assessment of the respiratory function is vital. A baseline should be established and used for comparison during future evaluations to monitor deterioration or improvement in function.

The comprehensive assessment of respiratory status includes x-rays to evaluate for rib fractures that may have occurred at the time of trauma; assessment of preexisting lung disease, such as chronic obstructive pulmonary disease or asthma; arterial blood gas studies to determine the balance of oxygen and carbon dioxide in the blood; and the vital capacity. Abnormal findings in any of these areas indicate that there is a compromised respiratory system and the patient may not be receiving adequate ventilation.

There are additional respiratory parameters that help the treatment team establish functional goals within the respiratory limitations of the patient. These parameters are vital capacity, tidal volume and respiratory rate; strength of the respiratory muscles, including the accessory muscles; breathing pattern in both supine and sitting positions (if possible); ability to cough and clear secretions; chest mobility; and the patient's posture. Upon admission and until the patient is medically stable, the respiratory parameters should be evaluated frequently.

VITAL CAPACITY

The vital capacity, the greatest amount of air that can be expired after a maximal inspiratory effort, may drop significantly within a few hours after injury. This may be due to a lesion that is progressing, an increase in spinal cord edema, or fatigue of the diaphragm.

Normal vital capacity measures 4 to 5 liters, although this may vary with height and weight differences. In a person with a spinal cord injury, vital capacity measurements are frequently less than 2 liters because of intercostal and abdominal muscle paralysis. If the vital capacity is less than 800 cc, mechanical ventilation is often necessary. Appropriate respiratory treatment, including deep breathing exercises, chest physical therapy, intermittent positive pressure breathing (IPPB), and muscle strengthening, lead to an improvement in vital capacity measurements.

The vital capacity measurement is frequently used clinically as an index of respiratory function. The value is important in determining if the patient can effectively move secretions from the alveoli to the airways. The greater the vital capacity, the greater the patient's ability to move secretions to the larger airways. The secretions can then be cleared from the airways by the patient's own ability to cough or by assisted coughing techniques.

Vital capacity measurements can be easily taken with a device such as a spirometer. The patient is instructed to take a deep breath and expel as much air as possible. Measurements should be taken frequently in the acute care phase and then on a weekly basis in the advanced stages of the rehabilitation program.

TIDAL VOLUME

Tidal volume is the amount of air that moves into the lungs with each respiration. Normal tidal volume is 0.5 liters, but may be decreased in a person with a spinal cord injury for the same reasons that vital capacity is reduced: loss of intercostal and abdominal muscle power. The tidal volume increases with improvement in the patient's vital capacity and also may be measured with a spirometer.

RESPIRATORY RATE

The respiratory rate should be assessed when the patient is at rest and unaware that his or her breaths are being counted. In an intact respiratory system, the respiratory rate is normally between 12 and 16 breaths/min. In a compromised respiratory system, often the respiratory rate is increased in an attempt to maintain adequate ventilation. The clinician should be alerted to the signs of hyperventilation and hypoventilation that may occur secondary to changes in the respiratory rate. Hyperventilation may cause feelings of faintness, tingling, or numbness in the extremities. Hypoventilation may result in drowsiness, irritability, or restlessness.

RESPIRATORY MUSCLE STRENGTH

Objective testing of respiratory muscle strength is often difficult in the early stages of recovery. A simple method of assessing diaphragm function is to observe the epigastric rise of the supine patient as he or she breathes deeply. When the diaphragm is contracting through the full excursion of the muscle, there is a contoured elevation in the epigastric area. When there is not a full epigastric rise and the patient is using the accessory muscles of inspiration, the normal elevation cannot be observed. This loss of epigastric rise indicates impaired diaphragmatic function.

In the early phases of management, standard manual muscle testing techniques cannot be used to evaluate neck and trunk muscle strength. The patient is not able to assume the traditional testing positions for these muscle groups, and the testing itself may stress the site of injury. Asking the patient to contract neck and abdominal muscles actively provides an adequate, although not completely accurate, assessment of the strength of these muscles.

Intercostal muscle strength is indirectly assessed by observation and measurement of chest expansion. Chest measurements are taken to evaluate the excursion of both the upper and lower rib cage. A tape measure can be used to record the measurements at the levels of the axilla and xiphoid process. Measurements of the excursion after maximal exhalation should be compared to the measurements following maximal inhalation. Normal chest expansion is 6.0 to 7.5 cm, but in a person with a spinal cord injury there may be a negative value. The negative value may be caused by paradoxical chest motion. This paradoxical motion is discussed below.

BREATHING PATTERN

The breathing pattern of the patient should be evaluated to determine the quality and quantity of the muscles' contribution to inspiration. A normal breathing pattern consists of rib elevation and thoracic expansion, and epigastric rise. When the diaphragm is weak, the accessory muscles of respiration may assist the diaphragm in ventilation, and the patient may demonstrate greater upper thoracic movement, rather than the normal epigastric rise.

Breathing patterns should be observed while the patient is in different positions as gravity may affect the muscles' efficiency, causing a change in the breathing pattern. For example, a supine position is a gravity-resisted position for the intercostal muscles during anterior chest expansion. However, this position allows the diaphragm to assume a more normal resting position and, therefore, better excursion. A sidelying position allows gravity to assist the intercostal muscles in anterior chest expansion. In a sitting position there may be an alteration in the patient's breathing pattern, especially if the abdominal muscles are weak or paralyzed. The resting position of the diaphragm changes because of the loss of support to the abdominal contents, and the muscle's efficiency is reduced.

Breathing patterns may change when the patient engages in activities, such as talking or eating, because they increase the need for ventilation. It is common to observe more activity in the neck accessory muscles during these activities.

Patients with cervical cord injury may exhibit a paradoxical breathing pattern, particularly when the diaphragm is the primary muscle of respiration that is intact. The paralyzed muscles of the thoracic cage passively collapse with inspiration when the diaphragm descends and expand with expiration when the diaphragm ascends. Because this is the reversal of the normal pattern of respiration it is considered to be a paradoxical breathing pattern and can be easily recognized when observing a patient from the side.

COUGH FORCE

The cough force should be evaluated to determine the patient's ability to clear secretions. Coughing is impaired when abdominal muscle function is decreased because the abdominal muscles provide the expulsive power necessary for a cough.

Coughs can be classified as *functional*, *weak-functional*, and *nonfunctional*. If the patient is able to produce secretions by means of a forceful cough, the cough is an effective, functional cough. If the patient is able to clear secretions from the airway, but cannot expel the secretions unless assisted with coughing, the cough is a weak-functional cough. If the patient is unable to inhale or exhale with any functional force and cannot move secretions out of the major airways, the cough is a poor, nonfunctional cough, and assistance will be required to clear secretions and cough.

CHEST MOBILITY

A mobile chest wall is extremely important for optimizing inspiratory capacity and lung expansion. If there is paradoxical rib motion because of intercostal muscle paralysis, the chest wall does not go through its normal excursion during respiration. Eventually the chest wall will lose its normal mobility, which will lead to further deficits in respiration.

Chest mobility may be assessed by using a tape measure to evaluate excursion in the same manner that is used to assess intercostal muscle function. Chest expansion should also be measured after an airshift maneuver. An airshift is a maneuver in which the patient inhales maximally, closes the glottis, relaxes the diaphragm, and allows the air to shift from the lower thoracic cavity to the upper thoracic cavity. An airshift maneuver may result in an increase in chest expansion of approximately 1.5 cm.

POSTURE

Because of poor respiratory reserve, a patient's posture affects his or her respiratory capacity. The effects of gravity and positional changes on the diaphragm and intercostal muscles have been previously addressed. The position and stabilization of the trunk should also be considered when assessing a patient's respiratory function. The accessory muscles of respiration work more efficiently in expanding the chest wall when the trunk is adequately supported. The spine should be maintained as close to normal alignment as possible in order to place the ribs in the most advantageous position for excursion.

Intervention Strategies

Prophylactic respiratory treatment is a lifetime process. Communication and education between the health care provider, the patient, and family members are important in optimizing the patient's function. Goals need to be defined and coordinated to ensure a successful, comprehensive respiratory program.

The two primary goals are (1) to maintain adequate bronchial hygiene and (2) to develop an adequate coordination of breathing with functional activities. The components of the respiratory treatment program are described in detail below.

POSTURAL DRAINAGE

Regular turning is important for preventing stasis of secretions in dependent areas of the lung. Even minor changes in position not only assist with the patient's comfort but also prevent the accumulation of secretions. Within the limitations of orthopedic alignment and stabilization and of patient tolerance, *postural drainage* should precede percussion and vibration techniques. Appropriate positions in supine, sidelying, and prone, with head elevated or lowered, should be selected to mobilize secretions of specific lung segments by means of gravity.

CHEST PHYSICAL THERAPY

Manual techniques used to clear the chest are often referred to as "chest physical therapy" and include *vibration* and *percussion*. The purpose of vibration and percussion is to dislodge and mobilize secretions into the bronchial tree. Secretions are then expectorated or suctioned. If there are no contraindications, these techniques should be used in conjunction with postural drainage.

BREATHING EXERCISES

Specific breathing patterns are taught to ensure a balanced use of all available muscles and ventilation to all parts of the lung. The breathing exercises should begin with slow, relaxed diaphragmatic breathing and progress to breathing with manual resistance applied over the diaphragm. Eventually, weights should be placed over the upper abdominal area (for approximately 15 min per session) while the patient attempts to maintain good diaphragmatic excursion (Fig. 4.1). It is important that the weights are placed over the upper abdominal region and are not resting on the lower ribs.

Localized breathing exercises should be used, when possible, to ventilate isolated lobes of the lung and improve movement of the thoracic cage. Pressure should be applied by the therapist to appropriate areas of the chest wall as the patient attempts to expand the chest in these areas. Most patients with intercostal muscle paralysis are not able to perform localized breathing exercises.

Inspirometers should be used both to provide visual feedback of progress to the patient and to determine the efficacy of the treatment program (Fig. 4.2).

ASSISTED COUGHING TECHNIQUES

The best way to ensure bronchial cleansing and chest wall mobility is to incorporate assisted coughing techniques into the treatment program. In the acute phase of care when the patient is immobilized, is on bedrest, or has severely limited upper extremity strength, assistance is required to cough. One of the most common methods of facilitating a cough is to instruct the person who is assisting the patient

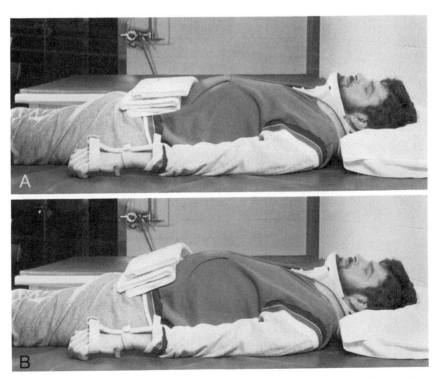

Figure 4.1. *A,* Weights on upper abdominal area for resisted diaphragmatic breathing. *B,* Diaphragmatic excursion with weights during deep inspiration.

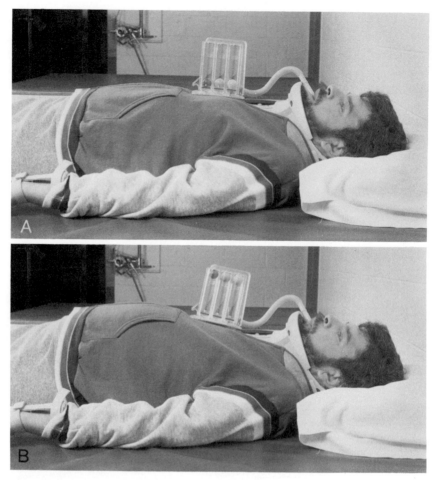

Figure 4.2. *A,* Incentive spirometer. *B,* Diaphragmatic excursion with incentive spirometer during deep inspiration.

to position his or her hand below the xiphoid process and to apply pressure into the abdomen with an inward and upward motion (Fig. 4.3). This motion should be coordinated with the patient's attempt to exhale forcefully. Some patients are able to position both of their hands below the xiphoid process and apply a quick inward and upward pressure while attempting to cough. This quick, compressive force simulates the contraction of the abdominal muscles. The manner of applying the pressure is similar to the Heimlich maneuver taught in cardiopulmonary resuscitation classes. This coughing technique is often referred to as the "quad cough."

Although it is easiest to perform this coughing technique in a supine position, it may also be done while the patient is in the sidelying or sitting positions. If the patient's sitting balance is stable, he or she may facilitate coughing independently by placing the hands over the upper abdominal area and quickly flexing the trunk forward when exhaling. Each patient should develop and modify the technique according to his or her level of ability and individual needs.

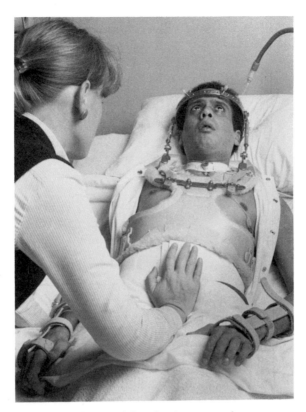

Figure 4.3. Quad assist cough.

CHEST MOBILITY

Treatment programs should be directed toward minimizing the range of motion deficits of the chest wall. If a joint does not have a sufficient range in which to move, any increase in strength will have little functional significance. Range of motion of the chest wall can be maintained or improved through deep breathing exercises, IPPB, assisted coughing techniques, passive manual stretching, and joint mobilization techniques. Airshift maneuvers can also improve chest wall mobility and should be taught to the patient.

In the rehabilitation phase of care, chest mobility is often facilitated by activities practiced during mat programs in physical and occupational therapy. For example, the trunk rotation that a patient uses to facilitate rolling to the sidelying or prone positions also stretches the chest wall. Any increase in the patient's activity level not only aids in maintaining good chest wall mobility but also assists with mobilizing secretions and enhances deep breathing.

POSTURE

Proper posture promotes better breathing, optimizes chest excursion, and improves vital capacity. Any abnormal posture, such as kyphosis or scoliosis, hinders rib and diaphragm movement.

A wheelchair that is fitted properly should provide adequate support for the patient. Occasionally, trunk supports may be needed to provide for postural alignment and stabilization of the trunk. Good alignment and stabilization help improve the efficiency of the primary and accessory muscles of respiration.

ABDOMINAL SUPPORTS

With paralyzed or weakened abdominal muscles, a corset or abdominal binder may be worn to support the abdominal contents against the effects of gravity. These supports allow the diaphragm to assume a better resting position while the patient is sitting upright.

Proper application and fit of the corset or binder are essential for adequate support. The corset/binder should lie over the lower (floating) ribs and extend over the iliac crests bilaterally. The lower portion of the corset should be tighter than the upper portion. Improper placement of the corset impedes epigastric rise and diaphragm function. The patient should be weaned from the corset as he or she adjusts to the greater respiratory demands of an upright position and an increased activity level.

Care of the Ventilation-Dependent Patient

CONSIDERATIONS FOR VENTILATORY SUPPORT

A patient who has sustained a high spinal cord lesion (C1–3) with paralysis of the diaphragm muscle requires immediate resuscitation and life-long ventilatory support. Mechanical ventilation may also be indicated when (a) there is deterioration in respiratory status from ascending edema in a lower cervical spinal cord injury, (b) there is unilateral diaphragm paralysis that may lead to extreme fatigue during times of greater respiratory demands, or (c) when quadriplegia occurs in elderly patients who have a history of respiratory system disease, such as asthma or chronic obstructive pulmonary disease.

Approximately one in ten patients who are placed on a ventilator will remain on it for a lifetime. For the rest, as the strength of the remaining respiratory muscles improves, the weaning process should be initiated. Prolonged mechanical ventilation should be avoided whenever possible to minimize the associated potential complications. These complications include infection, excessive secretions, pneumothorax, gastrointestinal complications, and necrotic changes in the trachea resulting from prolonged pressure from the tracheostomy tube and cuff. In addition, the communication difficulties associated with mechanical ventilation are extremely frustrating for the patient, family, and staff.

TYPES OF MECHANICAL VENTILATORS

The most commonly used ventilators are described as either "pressure-controlled machines" or "volume-controlled machines." The pressure-controlled or positive pressure-cycled ventilator operates by terminating the inspiratory phase of operation when a predetermined pressure is reached. Ideally, preset pressure should deliver the desired volume of gas to the patient. The volume-cycled machine operates by terminating the inspiratory phase of operation when a predetermined amount of gas is delivered to the patient.

The volume-cycled ventilator is more desirable for the patient with spinal cord injury. If the patient is unable to maintain a clear airway because of secretion retention, the desired volume of gas is still delivered to the patient in the volume-cycled machine. In the pressure-cycled ventilator, however, airway secretions may cause premature and rapid attainment of the preset pressure that terminates the inspiratory phase before the desired volume of gas can be delivered to the patient. Consequently, it may be extremely difficult to monitor the actual volume of gas that the patient is receiving with a pressure-cycled ventilator.

ARTIFICIAL AIRWAYS

An artificial airway is necessary when there is an upper airway obstruction, an interference of airway patency secondary to copious secretion retention, and/or when mechanical ventilation is utilized. Both the dysfunction and the anticipated length of time the patient is expected to be intubated determine what type of airway will be selected for management. The artificial airway may be sustained by either nasotracheal intubation or tracheotomy.

Nasotracheal Intubation. Nasotracheal intubation is selected for emergency situations or short-term intubation. The nasotracheal tube extends from the nose to the trachea. The intubation is poorly tolerated by the patient, and it often induces retching, vomiting, and excessive saliva formation. Communication is obviously impaired with nasotracheal intubation.

Tracheotomy. A tracheotomy is performed if the patient requires permanent mechanical ventilation or long-term ventilator assistance. A disposable plastic-cuffed tracheostomy tube or a reusable uncuffed metal tracheostomy tube must be inserted during an operative procedure. As with all operative procedures, there may be associated complications; these include tracheal trauma, infection, hemorrhage, and airway obstruction.

However, there are advantages in selecting a tracheotomy versus nasotracheal intubation for airway maintenance that may outweigh the possible complications of the surgical procedure. Of primary importance is the patient's comfort. A tracheotomy permits the patient to eat and communicate with less difficulty. In addition, secretion removal is facilitated through the tracheostomy tube.

EARLY MANAGEMENT OF THE VENTILATOR-DEPENDENT PATIENT

The entire treatment team is involved with the patient at the very early stages of management. It is important to establish a basic verbal and nonverbal communication system with the patient, family, and staff members.

The treatment program, although limited while the patient is on the ventilator, should include chest physical therapy, postural drainage, and suctioning within medical, surgical, and orthopedic limitations. The program should also include strength training of the accessory muscles of respiration.

Upper and lower extremity range of motion exercises should begin at bedside. Until the patient is surgically stable or is medically cleared for an increased activity level, upper extremity range of motion of shoulder flexion and abduction should be limited to 90° to avoid any undue stress to the fracture site. In addition, attention should be directed to proper positioning and pressure relief techniques to avoid skin breakdown while in bed.

When the patient is ready for an increase in activity level, elevation activities should be initiated, progressing gradually from an upright position in bed to lying in a reclining wheelchair (Fig. 4.4). A corset or abdominal binder is recommended when the patient begins upright activities.

The blood pressure and respiratory rate should be monitored for signs of hypoxia, postural hypotension, or respiratory distress. Respiratory distress may be indicated by tachycardia and/or tachypnea. Tachycardia is an increase in heart rate greater than 20 beats per min over the normal rate. Tachypnea is an increase in respiratory rate greater than 30 breaths per min over the patient's normal rate. Any abnormalities in these findings may indicate that the patient is adjusting poorly to the change in activity level, and the program must be revised accordingly.

Pressure relief techniques that were initiated while the patient was in bed should be continued as the patient increases the time out of bed in a chair or wheelchair. Weight shift techniques should be done at least every 20 to 30 min. During this phase of care, the patient

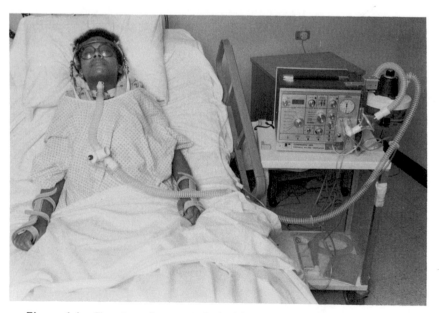

Figure 4.4.   Elevation of patient in bed while using a portable ventilator.

requires assistance from staff or family members to relieve pressure. (For additional information regarding pressure relief rationale and techniques, see Chapter 6.)

Use of a portable ventilator gives the patient an opportunity to leave the room either for therapy or for peer interaction. In the case of a medical emergency or equipment failure, a manual ventilator (i.e. AMBU® bag) and suctioning equipment should be transported with the patient at all times.

WEANING PROCESS

Patients on ventilator assistance require gradual withdrawal or weaning from ventilator support. The gradual process gives the patient time to strengthen the existing respiratory muscles in preparation for withdrawal of ventilatory support. Psychological preparation is also necessary for the patient who is learning to breathe without external assistance. The weaning process is often a time of high anxiety for the patient who previously had to depend on a machine to sustain life.

The weaning process may be initiated when the patient has a vital capacity of at least 800 cc and is free from infected secretions, water imbalances, or other uncontrolled pulmonary or medical complications.

There are two methods of ventilatory support commonly used during the weaning process: (1) a combination of assist control (AC) ventilator support and use of a T-piece (Fig. 4.5) and (2) intermittent mandatory ventilation (IMV) with or without use of a T-piece. The T-piece is used to provide humidification and oxygen to the patient, but does not provide any ventilatory assistance.

When using the AC method, the patient initiates the breath or triggers the ventilator for inspiration and then receives a preset volume of air. This method requires very little diaphragm effort to trigger the ventilator, and the diaphragm does not have to work at a constant level to maintain ventilation. *The AC method is the recommended method of ventilatory support for the person with a spinal cord injury.*

The IMV method allows the patient to initiate the breaths, but the IMV mode only delivers the amount of air that the patient initiates with voluntary inspiration. The diaphragm has to work constantly to

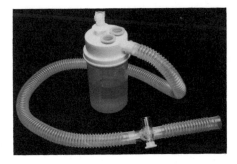

Figure 4.5. T-piece (adaptation to allow oxygen and moisture to flow across the tracheostomy site).

maintain adequate ventilation and does not receive a rest period. This method is not conducive to strengthening the diaphragm muscle and therefore often results in a failure to wean from mechanical ventilation.

If the patient experiences no difficulty tolerating the weaning process, the time off the ventilator, using only the T-piece, should be gradually increased. Initially, the T-piece should be used for four 5-min periods per day. The time should be increased as the patient's endurance improves. When the patient is weaned from the ventilator in this manner, the diaphragm does maximal work for short periods of time. If the patient is using the AC method of ventilatory support, the diaphragm has a rest period when the patient is placed back on the ventilator. In contrast, the IMV method does not allow a true rest and recovery period for the diaphragm when the patient is placed back on the ventilator.

Throughout the weaning process from ventilator support, the treatment program should continue as initiated in the ventilator-dependent phase of care. In addition, the patient should be instructed in deep breathing exercises, assisted cough techniques, and use of the incentive spirometer (using a nonfenestrated inner cannula tracheostomy attachment).

The patient should be transferred to a reclining wheelchair when he or she is able to tolerate the upright position in bed. The T-piece with a portable oxygen tank should be used for activities outside the patient's room. In the early stages of the weaning process, a manual ventilator (AMBU bag) and suction machine should accompany the patient at all times.

The goal of the weaning process is to have the patient attain complete withdrawal of ventilator support. Each patient must be evaluated on an individual basis. Some patients can not tolerate breathing without the ventilator throughout the entire day. Others may require rest periods when they are placed back on the ventilator.

After the ventilator support is withdrawn, the use of the T-piece should be gradually reduced and the tracheostomy removed. The process of withdrawing the T-piece and tracheostomy should begin when the patient can manage secretions and maintain acceptable blood gas levels on room air.

A small plug may be used to occlude the tracheostomy tube for intermittent periods of natural respiration and communication. The patient may only tolerate a few minutes of plug insertion every hour. As with all methods of accommodation, this time should be gradually increased until final tracheostomy extubation. Final extubation may be considered when the patient is able to clear secretions through the mouth, with or without assisted cough, and the vital capacity, vital signs, and blood gases are at acceptable levels.

Steps to reduce the stoma size should begin during the weaning process by using a progressively smaller tracheostomy tube that is changed every few days. The stoma will gradually heal, and the respiratory program should continue as described for non-ventilator-dependent patients.

ADDITIONAL TECHNIQUES OF BREATHING WITHOUT VENTILATOR SUPPORT

Patients who are ventilator-dependent may tolerate time off the support for short periods by using glossopharyngeal breathing (GPB) or "guppie" breathing. In this technique the patient uses the tongue, mouth, and throat to gulp air to the back of the throat and force it into the lungs. The patient must be comfortable on ventilator support and have normal tongue strength before learning GPB.

Electrophrenic nerve pacing may be used for the ventilator-dependent patient who has an intact phrenic nerve. A surgical procedure is required to implant the electrodes that stimulate the phrenic nerve, the innervation to the diaphragm. Electrophrenic pacing is usually not considered for the patient before 6 months following injury.

COMMUNICATION PROBLEMS

Communication is a major concern for the patient requiring mechanical ventilation and/or tracheostomy intubation. It is frustrating for the patient, family, and staff members if the patient cannot be understood when trying to communicate. The speech-language pathologist can be of invaluable assistance in providing the patient with appropriate mechanisms for communication.

There are several methods for facilitating communication with the patient on mechanical ventilation and/or tracheostomy intubation. These methods include the following:

1. Having the patient mouth the words slowly and enunciate as best as possible;
2. Using a language board that has phrases, pictures, symbols, and questions individualized for the patient's needs on one side (Fig. 4.6A) and the alphabet on the other side for quick scanning (Fig. 4.6B);
3. Deflating the cuff of the tracheostomy tube in order to allow air to flow around the tube and past the vocal cords; the volume from the ventilator may need to be increased to compensate for the air

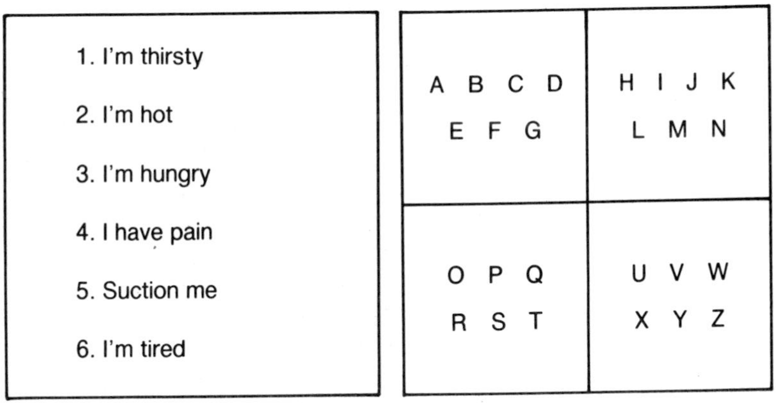

1. I'm thirsty	A B C D	H I J K
2. I'm hot	E F G	L M N
3. I'm hungry		
4. I have pain		
5. Suction me	O P Q	U V W
6. I'm tired	R S T	X Y Z

Figure 4.6. *A*, Basic needs language board. *B*, Blocked alphabet language board.

flowing around the tube. Physician permission is required for this method;

4. Using an electrolarynx—an artificial battery-powered device— while the patient attempts to talk. There are several types of electrolarynxes. The Western Electric device (Fig. 4.7A) may be held against the side of the neck while the patient mouths words. Another device is the Cooper Rand (Fig. 4.7B), which has a tube that is placed inside the mouth near the patient's cheek. It is also used to facilitate speaking. Use of the electrolarynx devices requires the assistance of another person because it is a hand-held device.

5. The Venti-Voice Communication Aid (TM) is designed to produce a tone pneumatically that is introduced into the patient's vocal tract through either a transnasal or oral catheter. It can be used while the patient is on the ventilator and is activated by the patient using a magnetic eyebrow switch.

A different mechanism of communication may be used for the patient who is using a T-piece during the weaning process. If the patient is able to be off the ventilator for at least an hour and has a fenestrated tracheostomy tube and a fenestrated inner cannula, an Olympic Trach Talk (OTT) may be used for communication (Fig. 4.8).

A fenestrated tracheostomy tube, a low-pressure, cuffed device with a removable inner cannula that exposes an opening on the outer cannula, allows the patient to talk during expiration. OTT is designed to fit over the fenestrated tube in the same manner as the T-piece. It has a valve that allows the patient to inhale through the tracheostomy tube. Upon exhalation, the valve closes, allowing the air to flow past the vocal cords and produce voice. The cuff of the tracheostomy tube must be deflated when using the OTT to permit adequate air flow. The patient can use this device without assistance.

Summary

The person who has suffered a cervical or high thoracic spinal cord injury is especially susceptible to respiratory complications. Pa-

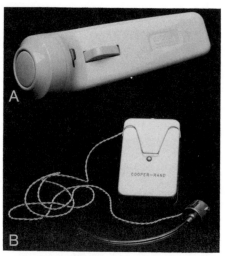

Figure 4.7.   A, Western Electric electrolarynx. B, Cooper Rand electrolarynx.

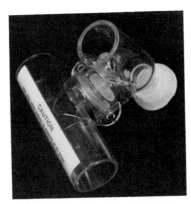

Figure 4.8. Olympic Trach Talk.

tient education is of paramount importance in the prevention and care of respiratory complications. A good respiratory program is an ongoing program that must be maintained throughout the lifetime of the individual.

Suggested Readings

Alvarez SE, Peterson M, Lunsford BR: Respiratory treatment of the adult patient with spinal cord injury. *Phys Ther* 61:1737–1745, 1981.

Ganong WF: *Review of Medical Physiology*, ed 8. Los Altos, CA, Lange Medical Publications, 1977.

Nixon V: *Spinal Cord Injury*. Rockville, MD, Aspen Systems Corporation, 1985.

Nursing 80 Photobook Series: *Providing Respiratory Care*. Horsham, Intermed Communication, Inc, 1979.

Zejdlik C: *Management of Spinal Cord Injury*. Monterey, CA, Wadsworth Health Sciences Division, 1983.

CHAPTER 5

Bladder and Bowel Management

CYNTHIA KRAFT, R.N., M.S.

Successful management of the person with a neurogenic bowel and bladder after spinal cord injury is crucial in enabling that person to return to a productive life in the mainstream of society. Neurogenic bowel and bladder management should being soon after injury in order to prevent the complications that may hinder the individual's progress through the rehabilitation program or increase his or her feelings of helplessness, frustration, and embarrassment.

The term "neurogenic" is used to describe a group of symptoms arising from neurologic rather than urologic pathology. Neurologic pathology may result in an absence of voiding, incomplete emptying of the bladder, inadequate storage of urine, absence of voluntary defecation, constipation, bowel incontinence, and/or intestinal obstruction.

Before looking at neurogenic bowel and bladder management, it may be helpful to review the normal anatomy and physiology of each of these systems. This brief review is followed by a discussion of how a spinal cord injury (SCI) affects each of these sytems, as well as management protocols.

Bladder

NORMAL ANATOMY OF THE GENITOURINARY SYSTEM

The kidneys produce urine as a by-product of filtering body fluids in order to conserve water and other substnces, maintain an acid-base balance, and both detoxify and excrete foreign, noxious, or nonessential elements. The urine is transported from the kidneys to the bladder by the ureters. At that ureterovesicle junction—that is, where the ureters enter the bladder—is a valve that assists in preventing backflow of the urine. Urine is stored in the bladder, which is a hollow organ composed of smooth muscle. At the neck of the bladder is the internal sphincter, which is a small muscle that has the function of closing off the bladder neck. Urine is transported from the bladder by the urethra, which is closed off by the external sphincter (Fig. 5.1).

NERVOUS CONTROL OF THE GENITOURINARY SYSTEM

Nervous system control of the genitourinary system is both voluntary and autonomic, involving the spinal cord and the brain. The spinal cord through S2–4 is responsible for providing the sensory input to the brain when the bladder is full. It is also responsible for the autonomic control of the internal sphincter. The brain (cerebral cortex, pons, and midbrain) is responsible for cerebral awareness of bladder fullness and control of the external sphincter.

Process Of Urination. Urination (micturition) is a coordination of voluntary and reflex actions to achieve both bladder contraction and sphincter relaxation. The act of micturition is a set of reflex activities coordinated through the brain. Inhibition or control of urination occurs within the cerebral cortex, midbrain, and pons.

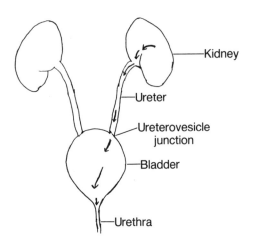

Figure 5.1.   Genitourinary system.

As the bladder sends out sensory impulses to the brain via the posterior columns and lateral thalamic tracts of the spinal cord, the individual becomes increasingly aware of the necessity to urinate. The brain signals the external sphincter whether this is an appropriate place and time to empty the bladder. If it is not, the sphincter remains closed.

HOW A SPINAL CORD INJURY AFFECTS THE GENITOURINARY SYSTEM

It is important to realize that a SCI can affect any part of urination, depending on the location and completeness of the injury. The length of time after injury also affects the clinical picture presented. Immediately after injury and for the first 3–6 weeks postinjury, the bladder is usually flaccid. Urinary retention results. Until bladder tone returns voiding that the individual may do is usually overflow incontinence. Overflow incontinence occurs when the amount of urine exceeds the bladder's capacity to contain it.

An injury to the spinal cord that results in an intact sacral arc (S2–4), a spastic paralysis, hyperactive deep-tendon reflexes, and hypoactive superficial reflexes is called an *upper motor neuron injury.* This type of bladder is called "reflex bladder." Any injury to the peripheral nerves—that is, occurring in the cauda equina region—results in a flaccid paralysis and a sacral arc that is not intact and is called a *lower motor neuron injury.* This type of bladder is an "areflexic bladder."

MANAGEMENT ROUTINES

Before instituting a bladder regimen for the neurogenic bladder, a complete urologic profile should be done to help ensure successful bladder management for the individual. A complete urologic profile is recommended on a yearly basis in order to help prevent genitourinary complications; it includes the following procedures:

1. *Urinalysis:* Tests are done for the pH, specific gravity, protein, casts, number of red blood cells, and number of white blood cells.
2. *Culture and sensitivity:* Tests are done for the type of bacteria and antibiotic sensitivity.
3. *IVP (intravenous pyelogram):* After injecting dye into the patient, a set of serial x-rays is taken to determine if there is normal functioning of the kidneys, ureters, and bladder.
4. *Cystourethrogram:* Dye is introduced into the bladder through a catheter. The catheter is clamped off, and an x-ray is taken to determine if reflux is present. The catheter is then removed, and the patient tries to void. If the patient is successful, another x-ray is taken to show the urethra and any abnormalities that may be present.
5. *Cystometrics (with urethral profile pressure):* The bladder is filled with gas through a catheter connected to a graphics machine. As the bladder fills, the pressure within it is recorded. As the catheter is slowly withdrawn, the pressure in the sphincter and urethra is also recorded.
6. *24-hr creatinine clearance:* All urine produced by the individual within a 24-hr period is collected and tested for the amount of creatinine contained in it. At the end of the 24-hr period, a blood sample is drawn. The ratio between the amount of creatinine in the blood versus kidneys is determined. Kidney function is determined by this comparison.

Other tests that may be ordered include a "KUB" (x-ray of the kidneys, ureters, and bladder) to determine the presence of stones; bladder EMG; a renal scan; or a renal ultrasound. The specific tests ordered may vary from physician to physician and from patient to patient.

Many factors need to be considered in a bladder management program. These factors include the individual's age, sex, previous medical problems, psychological status, discharge plans, and life-style. Ideally the patient should be informed about the various options in bladder management available to him or her and be able to choose the most practical, yet safe method.

Early Management. Immediately after injury, the most practical and safe bladder management is an indwelling catheter. The individual is given sufficient volumes of fluid in order to flush the kidneys and bladder and to assist in preventing symptomatic bacteriuria. A closed system of drainage should be used, with care being taken not to lift the drainage bag above the individual's body and to keep the catheter straight and free-flowing. The catheter should be changed according to hospital protocol, but at a minimum of every 30 days. Intermittent catheterization can be done during this period, but often, due to medical problems and the management of other problems, it is impractical and unsafe.

Postacute Management. Once medical stability has been achieved and the individual becomes more active, bladder management options should be addressed. As was stated previously, a complete urologic profile should be done. The individual should be informed of the options available and should be encouraged to participate actively to the extent that he or she feels comfortable in the bladder management program.

The options include (a) continued use of an indwelling catheter; (b) intermittent catheterization as part of a total bladder training program; and (c) a surgical diversion procedure, such as suprapubic cystostomy or ileal conduit.

Upper Motor Neuron Bladder.   In the male with an upper motor neuron bladder, the long-term goal in bladder management is a reflex emptying of the bladder with minimal postvoid residual. This is accomplished by using an intermittent catheterization program combined with limited, regulated fluid intake.

Fluid intake is restricted the night before the removal of the catheter. The Foley catheter is removed in the morning, the individual is placed on a 1800–2000 cc fluid restriction—400 cc at breakfast, lunch, and dinner and 200 cc at 10:00 AM, 4:00 PM, and 8:00 PM—and catheterization is scheduled every 4 hr. Limited fluid intake helps prevent overdistention of the bladder.

Just before each catheterization, the individual should be encouraged to try to manually stimulate the bladder to empty by tapping on the suprapubic area, stroking the inner thigh area, or gently pulling on pubic hairs. In order to avoid reflux of urine back into the kidneys, the crede maneuver should not be used on any individual with a reflex bladder. Should the individual void, he should be catheterized immediately with the voided volume and the catheterized volume carefully recorded.

Once the male patient has begun to void, an external catheter should be used to prevent the individual from getting wet between voiding. There are several commercially available devices with different methods of application. Each individual should be evaluated as to which type of external collecting device fits him best and best suits his needs. This evaluation may require some time and experimentation with different types of external catheters, as well as modes of application. It is often a frustrating time for the individual, and it should be explained to him that these feelings of frustration are normal.

As the bladder begins to empty on its own, reflexively, and/or when stimulated at appropriate intervals, the schedule of catheterization can begin to be tapered. Generally, consistent postvoid residuals of 50–100 cc indicate that the time interval between catheterizations can be increased. The individual should be encouraged to stimulate voiding between catheterization times in order to prevent overdistention of the bladder. In the ideal situation, the catheterization schedule can be totally eliminated.

Should the individual have difficulty voiding or emptying the bladder completely, various medications can be used to help stimulate the bladder emptying. Commonly used medication are phenoxybenzamine (Dibenzyline), bethanecol chloride (Urecholine), and baclofen (Lioresal). Dibenzyline's primary use in bladder management is to decrease internal sphincter tone. Urecholine is used to increase the strength of bladder contractions, thus forcing more urine completely out of the bladder. Lioresal is used to decrease bladder spasticity in order to allow greater filling capacity without reflexic emptying.

If the individual continues to have difficulty completely emptying his bladder over a period of time, a transurethral resection external sphincterotomy (TURES) should be considered. In this procedure, a portion of the elastic tissue at the neck of the bladder is removed, and an incision(s) is made in the external sphincter to decrease outlet resistance. One possible complication of the procedure is loss of the ability to have an erection. This is now prevented by avoiding the dorsal portion of the sphincter at the penile-scrotal junction when making the incision. However, a temporary loss of the ability to have an erection may be experienced for the first 4–6 weeks after the procedure. The individual must wear an external collection device at all times once the procedure is done because the bladder no longer has an obstructed outlet. Six weeks after the procedure is done, a cystometrogram with a urethral pressure profile should be done to check the effectiveness of the procedure.

Other options for long-term bladder management include the use of an indwelling catheter, either urethral or suprapubic. Although the indwelling catheter may not be considered the ideal medical management, certain factors may make it the best option for some people. If the individual has a high cervical injury and lacks a consistent, reliable primary caregiver who can do intermittent catheterization, an indwelling catheter may be the answer. Likewise if the individual needs long-term intermittent catheterization but because of an inability to void must remain on a fluid restriction, then potential medical complications, such as multiple urinary tract infections, pneumonia, and pressure sores, may necessitate the insertion of a catheter to allow the individual to consume large volumes of fluid without the fear of bladder overdistention. The most important consideration is what will work most realistically for that individual to make him as independent and functional as possible.

The choice of a urethral versus suprapubic catheter is not always an easy one for the individual to make. A urethral catheter comes from a natural orifice. It can remain in place or be removed for sexual intercourse. However, without proper taping of the catheter to the abdomen, a penile-scrotal fistula (see complications) may develop (Fig. 5.2).

A suprapubic catheter is surgically inserted directly into the bladder wall just above the symphysis pubis (Fig. 5.3). It is not a permanent procedure and is easily reversed by removing the catheter and allowing the site to close over. Closure will begin to occur within several hours after catheter removal, but the removal should be done with medical supervision. The advantages of a suprapubic catheter versus a urethral catheter are as follows:

1. A large catheter is used, making plugging less likely.
2. It is easy to change. Often, family members say that they consider it easier to change than a urethral catheter.

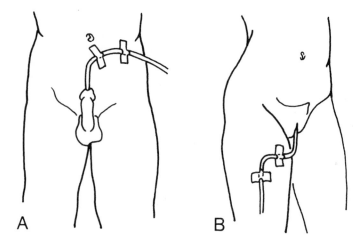

Figure 5.2.   A, Proper taping of an indwelling catheter (male). B, Proper taping of an indwelling catheter (female).

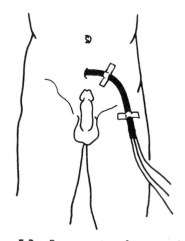

Figure 5.3.   Proper taping of a suprapubic tube.

3. It allows the spinal cord injured individual greater sexual freedom. Catheter removal and reinsertion are no longer of concern.
4. The individual will not develop a penile-scrotal fistula with a suprapubic catheter. Often, a suprapubic catheter is inserted as treatment for a fistula.

The disadvantages of a suprapubic catheter are

1. The catheter comes from a man-made orifice and may be considered "unnatural" by the individual and his family. It may take some time after the injury for the individual to be able to consider having the procedure done.
2. As with all surgical procedures, there are certain risks, albeit minor ones, connected with surgery. These should be explained to the individual by the urologist.

With an indwelling catheter, the individual must be able to consume 3–4 liters of fluid per day. Doing so helps naturally flush the kidneys and bladder and assists in preventing infections and the formation of stones. Other prophylactic care includes good hygiene, cleaning the penile-scrotal area with soap and water twice a day, cleansing of legbags and overnight drainage bags after each use, and taping the urethral catheter to prevent the development of a penile-scrotal fistula.

Most importantly, no matter what the bladder regimen, the individual and his caregiver(s) must be comfortable and knowledgeable in the care routine, management techniques, and the prevention of complications. Because of the emotional sensitivity surrounding bladder management, the individual should be encouraged to participate actively in decisions involving this area of care.

The female with an upper motor neuron bladder has different concerns than the male. Because of the unavailability of an adequate external collecting device for females, it is necessary to consider whether intermittent catheterization is practical for the individual— can she transfer from the wheelchair to the bed or commode, can she dress/undress herself, can she catheterize herself? If the answer to any of these questions is no, the practicality of intermittent catheterization must be reconsidered.

If the female with an upper motor neuron bladder does choose intermittent catheterization, the long-range goal is continence achieved by a limited fluid intake, frequent catheterizations, and timed voiding. The procedure for intermittent catheterization is the same as it is for males with an upper neuron bladder. Fluid intake is restricted to 1800–2000 cc per day, and catheterization is done very 4 hr. Should the individual void between catheterizations, it is important to determine if any one particular stressor triggers the incontinence. Some of the factors that may trigger the incontinence include (a) any specific activity, such as transfer; (b) urinary tract infection; (c) menstruation; and (d) a change in fluid intake.

Medications may need to be added to the regimen. Oxybutynin chloride (Ditropan) or pseudoephedrine hydrochloride (Sudafed) can be used to decrease bladder spasticity. Propantheline bromide (Probanthine) can be used to decrease spasticity, as well as problems with autonomic dysreflexia.

For some females, a urethral prosthesis may be the answer, rather than long-term intermittent catheterization. The urethral prosthesis is constructed to simulate the action of the sphincter and close off the urethra. It is made of two rods inserted on either side of the urethra, which are connected to a pressure device. The individual increases the pressure to closs off the bladder neck and decreases the pressure to open the bladder neck. Every individual should be evaluated carefully before being considered for the prosthesis.

The most common method of long-term bladder management for females with an upper motor neuron lesion is an indwelling Foley catheter. People have survived in a healthy state for many years with an indwelling catheter. However, of major importance to minimizing complications is the prophylactic care that the individual receives. The perineal area should be cleansed twice a day with soap and water. Fecal contamination should be avoided. The individual must be willing to drink 3–4 liters of fluid per day in an effort to flush the bacteria from the system. Legbags and overnight drainage bags should be cleansed after each use.

The size of the Foley catheter chosen should always be the smallest possible. Generally, no more than 16 french catheter should be used. The larger the catheter size, the more the urethra is stretched. A 5-cc balloon should be used to prevent the balloon from touching the bladder walls and causing erosion. Should leakage occur with an indwelling catheter, the individual should be instructed to add 1–3 cc of sterile water to the balloon after she has checked for catheter obstruction. If bladder spasticity remains a problem, the addition of Ditropan two to three times a day may be considered.

Lower Motor Neuron Bladder. In the management of the lower motor neuron bladder, the sex of the individual is usually not a consideration. Long-term goals and management principles remain the same: to prevent overdistention and promote adequate emptying of an infection-free bladder.

Because the lower motor neuron injury is an injury to the peripheral nerves, the paralysis experienced by the individual is a flaccid type with an atonic bladder that is unable to empty spontaneously. The voiding that is usually experienced is that of overflow incontinence with high postvoid residuals.

To begin the program of bladder retraining, the individual should be placed on a q 4 hr intermittent catheterization program with a fluid restriction of 1800–2000 cc. A record should be kept of each catheterization. When these volumes are consistently below 300 cc, the catheterization schedule may be changed to every 6 hr. It is expected that the individual is able to catheterize him- or herself because the extremities should be functional in a person with a lower motor neuron bladder.

After having a complete genitourinary workup, the individual may be taught to crede and/or be encouraged to strain in order to empty the bladder routinely. The individual should be taught the correct method of crede in order to prevent reflux and hydronephrosis. Nonforceful, smooth, even pressure should be applied over the bladder area beginning at the umbilicus and moving toward the symphysis pubis. Movement should be unidirectional. The individual may do this maneuver several times to empty the bladder completely.

If the individual continues on long-term intermittent catheterization, a simple, inexpensive, yet safe mode of catheterization management is the "clean technique." Ideally, the individual should be on an every 4–8 hr catheterization routine and should be independent in performing catheterizations.

Red rubber catheters or plastic catheters may be used in clean technique catheterizations. The individual should be instructed to wash the hands, as well as the area surrounging the urethral opening. The catheter should be lubricated and carefully inserted into the bladder. Once the bladder has been drained, the catheter should be removed, washed with soap and water, and stored in a clean place. The catheter can be reused until it is noncompliant or until the individual feels it should be replaced.

The person with SCI may at first be reluctant to try this method because of fear of increased infection. It should be explained that with frequent catheterizations bacteria are removed with the urine. Because the individual is performing self-catheterization, most of the bacteria that he or she may be introducing into the bladder is from his or her body or environment, and the body has built up antibodies to fight this bacteria effectively.

Clean technique may not be suitable for every individual and should not be done in the hospital where the risk of cross-infection is high, but it should be considered before discharge as a simple, inexpensive, yet safe method of bladder management.

Incomplete Injuries/Spinal Cord Syndromes. The individual who has an incomplete SCI may present a confusing clinical picture. Each individual must be evaluated independently, and a thorough genitourinary workup is essential in order to institute the most appropriate regimen.

Of equal importance, however, is the clinical picture each individual presents. Does he or she report awareness of bladder fullness or irritants? Are there complaints of urgency, frequency, pain, or burning on urination? Are any abdominal muscles physically able to work? Is the individual able to exert any muscular control over the urination?

There are no set protocols for management of this type of bladder. Often, a blending of management regimens, using basic principles of genitourinary hygience, is the most effective management routine.

COMPLICATIONS

The most common reason for rehospitalization of individuals with spinal cord injuries is the treatment of genitourinary complications. The incidence of many of these complications can be decreased if the individual and the primary caregiver pay close attention to genitourinary hygiene and care.

Urinary Tract Infection. The most common genitourinary complication in persons with SCI is urinary tract infection (UTI). This can be the result of many factors, including but not limited to frequent over distention of the bladder, poor fluid intake, incorrect catheterization technique, and dehydration.

Signs and symptoms of a UTI include fever, general malaise, nausea, vomiting, a sudden increase in spasticity, leakage between catheterizations, a change in bladder sensation, and sedimented malodorous cloudy urine. These symptoms are accompanied by an increased number of white blood cells in the urine and an increased white blood cell count.

The general rule for treatment of UTIs is to treat only symptomatic infections with antibiotics, i.e., do not treat routine urine culture results. Treatment with antibiotics should not begin until after a urine culture has been obtained, and then the individual may begin to receive treatment with a broad-spectrum antibiotic.

Individuals should also be instructed not to take aspirin or Tylenol to lower their temperature. Doing so only masks the fever and makes it more difficult to ascertain the problem. Instead, the individual should be instructed to increase fluid intake to at least 3 liters per day. If the individual is on a fluid restriction regimen, an indwelling catheter may need to be inserted temporarily to prevent bladder distention.

Bladder/Renal Calculi.   Bladder and renal calculi are a common complication for the spinal cord injured individual. Because the individual is often not bearing weight on his or her long bones, a demineralization of these bones occurs, with calcium being excreted through the kidneys. If the calcium is allowed to remain in the genitourinary tract long enough, calculi may form.

The signs and symptoms of bladder and renal calculi are very similar to those of a urinary tract infection. However, of particular importance is a sudden, severe increase in spasticity, leakage around a catheter, leakage between catheterizations, and an increase in sediment present in the urine. Of significance also is a history of calculi formation. Diagnosis of calculi is made through an IVP, renal scan, KUB, and/or cystoscopy. Treatment of calculi is usually done by surgical removal or crushing of the calculi.

Hydronephrosis.   Hydronephrosis is a dilation of the kidneys as a result of poor excretion. Often this is a result of reflux; urine is forced back up the ureters to the kidneys as a result of lower tract obstruction, increased intravesicle pressure, or faulty ureterovesicle valves. It can also result from calculi preventing the drainage of urine or chronic infections. Diagnosis and the extent of involvement are determined by IVP or renal scan.

In the most severe cases, an indwelling catheter should be reinserted, and fluids should be forced for 1–3 months. Intermittent catheterization should then be prescribed. If chronic infections are the suspected cause of the hydronephrosis, then long-term antibiotic treatment should be added to the regimen.

Penile-Scrotal Fistula.   A penile-scrotal fistula is a pressure sore at the penile-scrotal junction. It is usually caused by long-term use of an indwelling catheter in males without proper taping of the catheter to the abdomen. Proper taping of the catheter to the abdomen prevents pressure and friction at the junction, and the importance of doing this can not be overemphasized. Once a fistula has occurred, it is difficult to heal and remain healed.

The treatment for a penile-scrotal fistula is removal of the urethral catheter. Often, a suprapubic catheter is inserted in its place until healing occurs.

Autonomic Dysreflexia.   Autonomic dysreflexia is a vasomotor response to the noxious stimuli below the level of injury that occurs in individuals who have suffered an injury at T6 or above. In over 85% of cases, the cause of autonomic dysreflexia is bladder-related, either from overdistention, blocked catheter, overfilled drainage bags, a UTI, or stones.

The signs and symptoms of autonomic dysreflexia include sudden onset of a pounding migraine-like headache, severely increased blood pressure, flushing and diaphoresis above the level of injury, and goosebumps. Treatment for autonomic dysreflexia is removal of the cause. To avoid a hypotensive crisis blood pressure should be carefully monitored as the problem is slowly removed.

Bowel

NORMAL ANATOMY OF THE GASTROINTESTINAL SYSTEM

The gastrointestinal (GI) system starts with the mouth and teeth where food begins to be broken down and digested. Food is transported from the mouth to the stomach via the esophagus. In the stomach, it continues to be digested. It continues along the GI tract to the small intestine where the process of breaking down the food into nutritional and waste products is completed. Nutritional products are absorbed into the bloodstream, and waste products are transported into the large intestine. The large intestine absorbs water and makes the waste products into a more solid mass. The waste products are then transported to the sigmoid colon for storage before entering the rectum, passing through the internal sphincter, and then the external sphincter to the outside of the body.

NERVOUS CONTROL OF THE GASTROINTESTINAL TRACT

Nervous control of the GI tract is both voluntary and autonomic, involving the spinal cord and brain.

The spinal cord through S2–4 is responsible for sensory input to the brain, signalling the brain when the rectum is full after sensing that pressure is being exerted against the internal sphincter. It is also responsible for the autonomic control of the internal sphincter. The brain—cerebral cortex, pons, and midbrain—is responsible for cerebral awareness of a full rectum and voluntary control of the external sphincter.

Physiology of Defecation. Defecation requires the coordination of voluntary and reflex actions to achieve rectal emptying. The act of defecating is a set of reflex activities coordinated through the brain. Inhibition, or control of defecation, occurs within the cerebral cortex, pons, and midbrain. As the rectum sends out impulses signalling the brain of the need to empty, the individual becomes increasingly aware of the necessity to defecate. As the awareness increases, the brain signals the external sphincter whether it is an appropriate time and place to empty. If it is not, the sphincter remains closed. The process is illustrated in Figure 5.4.

HOW A SPINAL CORD INJURY AFFECTS THE GASTROINTESTINAL SYSTEM

It is important to realize that a SCI affects only the ability to empty the rectum once the initial effects of the injury have passed.

Any injury to the spinal cord that results in an intact sacral arc (S2–4), spastic paralysis, hyperactive deep-tendon reflexes, and hypoactive superficial reflexes is called an upper motor neuron injury and causes a "reflex bowel."

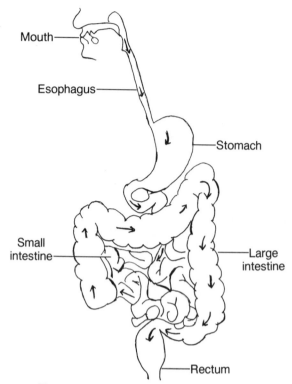

Figure 5.4. Gastrointestinal system.

Any injury to the peripheral nerves—that is, one occurring in the cauda equina region—results in a flaccid paralysis and a disrupted sacral arc and is called a lower motor neuron injury. The type of bowel caused by that injury is an "areflexic" or "flaccid" bowel.

MANAGEMENT ROUTINES

A good bowel program is one that (a) achieves results within a reasonable amount of time (one half-hour) and produces an adequate amount of stool with good consistency; (b) works by local stimulation, (i.e., digital stimulation and/or suppository); and (c) occurs at the same time of the day reliably, without accidents.

Before setting up any bowel routine, several factors need to be assessed. These include the following:

1. Premorbid habits: premorbid routine or pattern or bowel problems;
2. Diet: adequate nutritional intake or a major change in diet or eating patterns;
3. Fluid intake: adequate hydration to prevent constipation;
4. Activity level: level of ability and ability to sit up at 90°;
5. Level of injury;
6. Time elapsed since injury.

In order to set up an effective bowel program, all of these factors must be assessed and considered before implementation of the plan.

Early Management.   The first week to 2 weeks after injury, the most common GI problems are paralytic ileus and GI bleeding. Each of these problems should be addressed independently before considering long-term management of the neurogenic bowel.

When a state of atony of the small intestine exists with the absence of peristaltic movement, the individual is said to have a *paralytic ileus*. This complication usually occurs within the first 24 hr after injury and usually lasts about 1 week. The exact cause is unknown, although it might be the result of the sudden cessation of autonomic innervation. It occurs most commonly in cervical injuries.

Treatment of this complication is relatively simple—insertion of a nasogastric tube, aspiration of gastric contents, and connection to low suction until bowel sounds return. Also, the individual should remain NPO until bowel sounds return.

In approximately 5% of all persons with spinal cord injury GI bleeding occurs within the first 7–10 days after injury. Speculation is that it is either caused by an endogenous release of steroids in response to the injury, increased hydrochloric acid production from unopposed stimulation of the vagus nerve, and administration of steroids in an attempt to decrease swelling of the spinal cord.

Signs and symptoms of GI bleeding include heme-positive stools, an unexplained decrease in blood pressure, an increase in pulse rate, and a decrease in hematocrit and hemoglobin.

Many SCI centers are now placing individuals on prophylactic treatment soon after the injury occurs and are continuing medication for 3–6 months postinjury. Two drugs are presently being used: cimetidine (Tagamet) 300 mg four times a day and ranitidine hydrochloride (Zantac) 150 mg twice a day.

Postacute Management.   Once bowel sounds have returned, it is time to begin a bowel routine. With the resolution of an ileus in an individual with an upper motor neuron bowel, the defecation reflex returns, enabling the bowel to empty automatically. However, there is a loss of voluntary control. In an individual with a lower motor neuron bowel, the resolution of an ileus will mean the return of some intrinsic response of the smooth muscles in the bowel, but the defecation reflex is lost.

No matter what the level of injury, the individual should be encouraged to participate actively in setting up the program and evaluating it. The area of bowel control is often emotionally sensitive, and the individual's feelings should be acknowledged. Initially, participation of the person with a SCI may only involve reading informational material and providing premorbid information. With time, he or she may feel more comfortable with the area of bowel control, and increased participation should then be encouraged.

Many individuals who may be unable to perform the routine themselves may feel uncomfortable with having their spouse or parent perform it for them. These are not unnatural feelings and should be acknowledged as such. If possible, options for attendant care for this particular activity should be explored with the person.

Some general guidelines for setting up a bowel routine, no matter what type of injury the individual may have suffered, are as follows:

1. When at all possible, use premorbid patterns in scheduling the time of the routine. For example, if the individual always moved his or her bowels after dinner, schedule the program for the early evening;
2. Consider the type of activities the person will be doing after discharge. If the person is returning to school or work, a morning routine may be more feasible.
3. If there will be attendant care, schedule the bowel routine during that time.
4. Avoid the long-term use of harsh laxatives. They are not needed routinely if a routine is well established and will not cause rectal irritation, bleeding, or cramping.
5. When problems occur, evaluate all variables, looking for a change in one of them. For example, food that bothered the person before their injury will still be bothersome afterwards. The injury did not change that response.
6. Make one change at a time in the program. Allow some time before introducing another change.
7. Encourage patient participation in problem solving.
8. Not every individual moves the bowels daily, nor is it imperative that he or she does. Again, premorbid patterns may be helpful.
9. Medications should be kept to a minimum. Stool softeners and peristaltic stimulators can be used, but their usage should be evaluated individually. Often a change in dietary intake is equally as helpful.

The long-term goal of management of either type of neurogenic bowel is the same—a reliable program giving good results in a reasonable amount of time, occurring at the same time of the day, without incontinence.

Upper Motor Neuron Bowel. Management of the upper motor neuron bowel is based on using the defecation reflex. Local stimulation should be done after checking the rectum for hard stool. The hard stool should be carefully removed manually. Any soft stool should be removed by doing digital stimulation. In this procedure a gloved, lubricated finger is gently inserted into the rectum and moved in a circular, clockwise motion for 30–60 sec to stimulate rectal emptying.

Generally, the individual is started on a Dulcolax suppository every other day. It should be inserted past the sphincter and placed against the wall of the bowel. After 10–15 min digital stimulation can be done to assist in moving the stool. If the individual is able to sit at 90°, he or she should be placed on the toilet or a commode chair to allow gravity to assist the elimination.

A record should be kept of when the bowel routine is done, the amount of time it takes to achieve results, the consistency and amount of stool, and any incontinence. By doing this, it is easy to determine patterns that may be developing, as well as any problem areas. For example, if it is taking several hours for the individual to have results, it might be worthwhile to try a Fleet Bisacodyl Enema instead of the Dulcolax suppository. The suspension of the medication in a small amount of liquid instead of in suppository form has also been effective in alleviating this problem.

If the individual has previously not been able to sit up on the commode chair, the bowel program may be more effective and faster when he or she is able to do so. If the individual is incontinent on the days in which a suppository is not inserted, a program of daily suppository usage may be needed.

The best way to solve problems with an individual's routine is with the participation of that individual! Unless the program is reliable and realistic, follow-through after discharge is unlikely and the person may end up with problems.

Lower Motor Neuron Bowel.   The management of a lower motor neuron bowel is much more difficult because of the loss of the defecation reflex. The individual with a lower motor neuron bowel may often experience bowel incontinence because of flaccid internal and external sphincters and may be fearful that this problem may never be alleviated.

Initially, the individual should be placed on a daily suppository program. Hard stool should be manually removed. Digital stimulation will not accomplish any results in this type of injury and so is unnecessary. The suppository should be placed against the bowel wall. Twenty min after insertion, a rectal check should be done. If stool can be felt, the individual should be transferred to a commode chair. He or she should then be encouraged to try to push the stool out.

With some individuals, it might be reassuring to do a rectal check at the other end of the day, in order to be assured that no stool is present in the lower rectum. This rectal check can be eliminated as the individual gains more confidence in him- or herself and the program.

COMPLICATIONS

The most serious GI complications that the person with SCI can experience are diarrhea, impaction, and autonomic dysreflexia.

Diarrhea.   Diarrhea in the spinal cord injured individual is usually caused by one of three factors: (1) liquid stool being pushed past an impaction, (2) food or medication irritant, or (3) a virus. Depending on other factors presented with the diarrhea, it is usually easy to narrow down the cause. If there is any question that an impaction may be the cause, a flat plate of the abdomen should be considered to rule this out.

Treatment of diarrhea is usually symptomatic. An increase in fluid intake should be recommended to replace the fluids lost through the stool.

Impaction.   When the bowel becomes impacted, it is imperative that the stool be removed as expediently as possible. Signs and symptoms of impaction are nausea, vomiting, loss of appetite, feeling bloated, distended abdomen, poor or no results from a bowel program for several consecutive days, decrease in bowel sounds, and small amounts of liquid stool. Diagnosis is usually made with a flat plate of the abdomen.

Treatment consists of removing the impaction. Because the stool is usually higher up than a prepackaged enema can reach, treatment is usually given by mouth. Several medications can be given, including Dulcolax tablets, or a milk of magnesia and mineral oil cocktail. The use of large-volume enemas is contraindicated because of the danger of eliciting the crisis of autonomic dysreflexia. It is important to continue treatment until the bowel has been cleared of stool. After this has been accomplished, a bowel regimen should be reinstituted and assessed carefully to prevent this problem from recurring.

Autonomic Dysreflexia. Autonomic dysreflexia is a vasomotor response to a noxious stimulus below the level of injury that occurs in individuals who have suffered an injury at T6 or above. (See the discussion on neurogenic bladder complications for its signs and symptoms.) Although in over 85% of cases it occurs as a result of bladder stimuli, it can occur as a result of an overdistended rectum. If this is the cause, treatment should consist of insertion of a Nupercaine cream, waiting for 10 min, and then gentle manual disimpaction of the rectum.

Conclusion

The successful management of neurogenic bowel and bladder may not be an easy task; however, it is one that can be successfully done. When the person with SCI gains confidence and is secure in the management routine, he or she is more able to re-enter the mainstream of society and particpate fully in vocational, social, and sexual activities without the fear of embarrassing incontinence.

Suggested Readings

Barry K: Neurogenic bladder incontinence. *Rehab Nurs:* 12–13, 1981.

Hanak M, Scott A. *Spinal Cord Injury; An Illustrated Guide for Health Care Professionals.* New York, Springer Publishing Co, 1983, pp 66–100.

Hardy AG, Elson R: *Practical Management of Spinal Injuries.* New York, Churchill Livingston, 1976, pp 103–128.

Koff SA, Diokno AC, Lapides J: Neurogenic bladder dysfunction. *Am Fam Prac* 19:100–109, 1979.

Staas WE, DeVault PM: Bowel control. *Am Fam Prac:* 7:90–100, 1973.

Staas WE, LaMantia JG: Bowel function and control. In Ruskin AP (ed): *Current Therapy in Physiatry.* Philadelphia, WB Saunders, 1984, pp 405–410.

Staas WE, LaMantia JG: The neurogenic bladder: Physiologic mechanisms and clinical problems of bladder control. In Ruskin AP (ed): *Current Therapy in Physiatry.* Philadelphia, WB Saunders, 1984, pp 396–405.

CHAPTER 6

Pressure Sores: Prevention and Management

DEBORAH A. NAWOCZENSKI, M.Ed., P.T.

Pressure sores, commonly known as decubitus ulcers, are one of the most frequent problems following spinal cord injury (SCI) and one of the major causes of hospital readmission. They account for 7–8% of the deaths among the population with SCI. Pressure sores are not only an unnecessary complication but also one of the most costly. Conservative estimates of the cost per lesion approaches $30,000, and statistics from the National SCI Data Research Center indicate that the cost of hospitalization increases five-fold if a pressure sore (those greater than a Grade II) is serious enough to require plastic surgery.

In addition to the economic costs of pressure sores there are the vitally important social costs that affect both patient and family members. Pressure sores cause disruption to the family unit and time away from employment. Debilitating effects, such as loss of function, strength, and endurance, result when a person's mobility level has to change in attempts to heal these lesions.

The prevalence of pressure sores is determined by the physiologic intactness of the spinal cord. It is estimated that 60% of patients who sustain complete cervical spine injuries and 40% who suffer incomplete injuries will develop pressure sores; half of this population will have multiple sites of involvement. The paraplegic population is slightly overrepresented in the prevalence of pressure sores, with 50% of the population with complete injuries and 30% with incomplete injuries developing skin breakdown. The paraplegic person with an incomplete lesion generally develops a single site of involvement. More often, the person with a complete SCI often has multiple sites of pressure sore development, the most frequent site being the gluteal-sacral region. The trochanter and ischial regions closely follow in frequency of the development of skin breakdown.

With the establishment of Model SCI Centers in the United States, early admission to a definitive system has been shown to be a significant factor in reducing the prevalence of pressure sores. There is a considerably higher prevalence of skin breakdown in patients admitted to a SCI Center more than 72 hr postinjury as compared to patients admitted less than 72 hr after injury. It is felt that the specialized, rapid transport of acutely injured SCI individuals and the availability of expert professionals play a major role in the decreased prevalence of pressure sores in patients admitted to an SCI Center immediately after injury.

The morbidity and mortality of pressure sores are clearly significant, and prevention is the primary goal. Prevention, however, depends on a thorough understanding of the etiology of pressure sores.

Etiology

The primary factors associated with skin breakdown are pressure and time. Pressure may be defined as the force per unit area. If the forces on an area of the body are great enough for a long enough duration, capillary blood flow is obstructed, blocking cellular metabolism and leading to tissue necrosis. If the forces developed are concentrated in a very small area, then even greater pressure is generated in this area. Intense pressures applied for short durations may be as damaging as lesser pressures applied for prolonged periods of time. Furthermore, higher pressures are developed on the perimeter of a wound than within the wound itself. When the applied pressure exceeds normal capillary pressure—ranging from 14 mm Hg on the venous side to 35 mm Hg on the arterial side—tissue injury results. Microscopic changes may occur in the skin in only 1 hr of continuous pressure of 60 mm Hg! Actual pressure necrosis can develop with a continuous pressure of 300 mm Hg whether tissue is normal or denervated.

A SCI causes an alteration of the vasomotor pathways with a loss of vasomotor tone. Circulation to the muscles, skin, and mucosa is affected, further compromising blood flow to the tissues. Poor oxygenation to the tissues, poor cell nutrition, and a decrease in venous return result. Orthostatic edema develops with an increased accumulation of interstitial fluid. An increase in pressure to an area that is vascularly compromised only accelerates the progression of tissue necrosis.

Other primary factors lead to skin breakdown, including *direct pressure, shearing forces,* and *skin maceration. Direct pressure* is pressure unrelieved by turning or weight shifting and also pressure caused by forces of trauma, such as those incurred during transfers or mat activities. A poorly fitting wheelchair, clothes, or shoes may also cause direct pressure on an area of skin.

Pressure sores may be secondary to *shearing forces* imposed on the skin as one surface slides over another. Sliding down in bed with bed changes, poor turning and transfer techniques, and sliding rather than lifting all increase shearing forces. Spasticity may augment the effect of shearing forces as it may cause the limbs to slide repeatedly across a surface or press directly against another part of the body for a prolonged period of time.

Maceration, resulting from prolonged contact with urine, feces, sweat, or the combination of those substances, is directly related to the development of skin breakdown. A warm, moist environment is an optimal medium for bacterial growth, and skin that is softened by constant moisture is less resistant to the forces of direct pressure and friction than skin that is dry.

Other causative factors are associated with the formation of pressure sores. These factors include *sensory* and *motor loss, temperature changes,* and *chronic infections.*

With the loss of afferent (sensory) pathways, the patient cannot feel the discomfort resulting from pressure on an area and therefore is unaware of the need for a position change. If there is continued pressure, ischemia and tissue death result. Even with intact sensory input, impaired motor pathways interfere with the patient's ability to change position physically.

Temperature increase is a factor of concern in skin breakdown. A rise of 1.0°C in skin temperature causes a 10% increase in tissue metabolism and an equal increase in oxygen demand to tissues that are already compromised vascularly. It creates a situation in which "demand" exceeds the "supply" of available nutrition and oxygenation. Consequently, breakdown follows.

Chronic systemic infections, such as urinary tract infections, respiratory tract infections, and infections secondary to existing pressure sores, directly affect tissue nourishment and delay tissue healing. In addition to compromising the general health of the individual, systemic infections are usually accompanied by a rise in body temperature. The rise in body temperature causes the same effect on tissue metabolism as occurs with a local increase in skin temperature.

Psychosocial factors have been related to the incidence of pressure sores. In general, satisfaction with life activity—employment, avocational activities, living arrangements, and sexual activities—is closely correlated with the presence or absence of skin problems and a person's attitude toward the importance of skin care. A person who is satisfied with his or her life activity and feels strongly about the importance of skin care generally experiences fewer "interrupted" days of normal daily activities than the individual who is dissatisfied with his or her present life situation.

The nutritional status of the patient has an important effect on the maintenance of tissue vitality and wound healing. Maintaining proper nutrition is often a problem following SCI. A number of variables can affect a patient's nutritional status; they include a *negative nitrogen balance, anorexia, obesity, and repeated infections.*

Negative nitrogen balance frequently occurs following trauma and contributes to weight loss and tissue wasting. This condition is further aggravated if a person should become anorexic following SCI and loses additional adipose tissue coverage. Bony areas become prominent, thereby increasing the forces per unit area. A protein deficiency that usually occurs with a negative nitrogen balance may be compounded by the loss of protein from an existing infected ulcer.

Obesity not only impairs an individual's ability to perform activities of daily living but may also interfere with the ability to perform pressure-relief techniques. In addition, such equipment as a wheelchair or braces may no longer fit the patient who has gained excessive weight, and skin breakdown may develop in high-pressure areas.

Prevention and treatment of pressure sores require a team effort with close communication among the members so that appropriate methods of management can be maintained without compromising other facets of the patient's care. *The patient must be the most knowledgeable and directive member of the rehabilitation team.* Repeated emphasis must be placed on the cornerstone of management: prevention.

Changes Associated with Abnormal Pressures

HISTOLOGIC CHANGES

Histologic changes are associated with ischemic necrosis. In a normal response to direct pressure, the superficial capillary loops beneath the epidermis are compressed, and blood is immediately expressed from the area. Following removal of temporary compression an excess of blood flow to the area occurs within seconds. There is dilation of the small vessels reacting to chemical stimuli from the accumulation of metabolic products during the time of circulatory compression. An area of local redness from this response will usually disappear in 3–20 min.

Following prolonged ischemia, local inflammation of the tissues occurs. Arteriolar dilation, the first event to occur upon removal of pressure, results in an increase in the amount of blood that accumulates in the capillaries, as well as a rise in intercapillary volume and pressure. These actions, together with the infiltration of some cell mediators that directly affect the injured capillary walls, lead to extravasation of fluid into the interstitial tissues.

As the tissue edema increases, the metabolic exchange of nutrients, carbon dioxide, and oxygen becomes less efficient. Tissue death occurs due to anoxia and chemical injury from accumulation of catabolic products. The degree of tissue damage is related to the duration of the ischemic episode.

As the margin between living and necrotic tissue becomes clearly demarcated, an ulcer develops. Necrotic tissue becomes dehydrated and blackened in contrast to the surrounding skin, which becomes inflamed. It is important to note that underlying tissue death precedes the appearance of superficial ulceration. Ulceration is usually delayed for a period from 3 to 18 days before the patient or clinician notices broken skin or exudate from an open area.

CLINICAL CHANGES

In addition to the internal changes that occur with pressure, there are observable clinical changes as well. When pressure is initially applied to an area on the skin, blanching occurs as blood is expressed from the area. When the pressure is removed, blood immediately returns to the area indicating that the reflex arc of dilatation is in effect. It is a reactive hyperemic response, and the redness lasts for approximately 50% of the time that the pressure had been applied. This is a normal response to temporary pressure.

If there is prolonged pressure over an area, there may be a localized inflammatory response with the formation of edema. When this area is pressed by the examiner, blanching may or may not occur. If blanching remains after pressure is removed, the normal reflex arc of dilatation is not in effect, which is indicative of tissue necrosis. There is usually localized warmth, a possible blister, or a bluish discoloration in the area. Swelling or small lumps may be palpable. The person must not put pressure on the area until the signs of pressure are reversed. If the causative factors are not removed, then an ulceration will develop.

CLASSIFICATION OF PRESSURE SORES

Pressure sores are classified as Grade I, II, III, and IV according to the system developed by the National Spinal Cord Injury Data Collection System.

Grade   I: Limited to superficial epidermis and dermal layers;

Grade II: Involving the epidermal and dermal layers and extending into the adipose tissue (Fig. 6.1);

Grade III: Extending through the superficial structures and adipose tissue down to and including muscle (Fig. 6.2);

Grade IV: Destroying all soft tissue structures down to bone, with communication with bone or joint structures or both (Fig. 6.3).

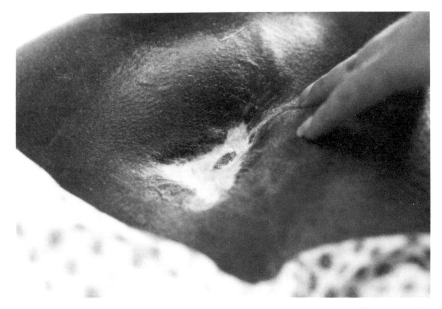

Figure 6.1.   Grade III pressure sore involving the epidermal and dermal layers of the skin.

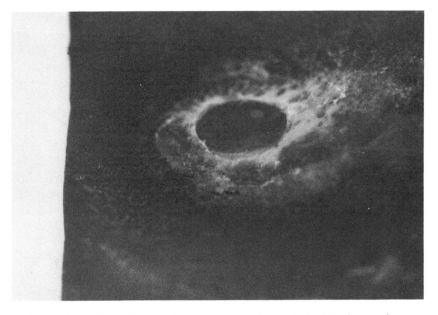

Figure 6.2.   Grade III pressure sore extending (and including) to the muscle.

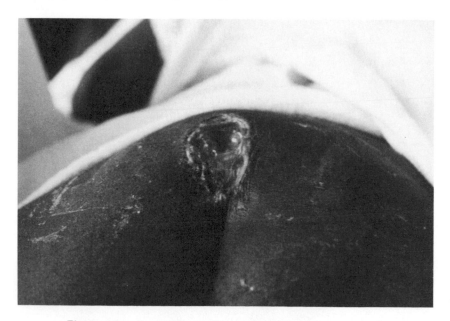

Figure 6.3.   Grade IV pressure sore extending to the bone.

KEY AREAS OF BREAKDOWN

Key areas of skin susceptible to breakdown are depicted in Figure 6.4. The bony prominences have been identified because they carry the greatest forces on their very small surface areas while the individual is in a supine, prone, sidelying, or sitting position. Table 6.1 lists the most common sites of pressure sores, positions where they most likely develop, and activities or forces that may contribute to breakdown. The list is not exhaustive and should only be used as a guide for the health care team member in the prevention and protection of the skin.

Prevention, Protection, and Intervention Strategies

As previously mentioned, the key to pressure sore management is prevention. Prevention is a 24-hr-a-day process. All patient educational programs should be directed toward prevention and should include physicians, nurses, therapists, attendants, and family members. Most importantly, the onus of responsibility must lie with the person who is spinal cord injured.

REMOVING OR MINIMIZING THE SOURCE OF PRESSURE

The primary method of relieving pressure is to remove the source of pressure. Correct positioning in bed is important, and all bony prominences should be supported in a manner that relieves forces over small surfaces and distributes forces evenly over large surface areas. In the acute phase, the initial recommended patient-turning schedule in bed is a quarter-turn every 2 hr. This schedule should be

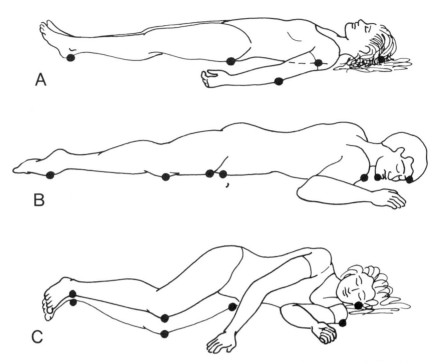

Figure 6.4. Key areas of skin breakdown in A, supine; B, prone; and C, sidelying positions.

adhered to regardless of what type of bed is used in the facility. As a person's skin tolerance improves, the amount of time spent in one position should be increased gradually. Skin inspection should always follow an increase of time in one position or after a person assumes a new position, such as sitting in a wheelchair for the first time. If the normal hyperemic responses can be elicited, then the time may be increased for that position. A general guideline to follow is to increase time in one position 15 min before changing position.

Instructions in pressure relief techniques should be provided to the patient and family as soon as possible following injury and should be reinforced consistently by the entire health care team. As much effort as possible should be made by the patient to relieve pressure while in bed by turning or by reminding others to turn him or her.

After the acute phase of care, when a person with a spinal cord injury is able to tolerate wheelchair activities, pressure relief techniques in the chair are equally important for prevention of skin breakdown. If the patient has the motor ability and balance to execute a "push-up" while in the wheelchair, then this activity serves a dual purpose: relieving pressure and maintaining strength in the upper extremities. A wheelchair push-up is accomplished by locking the elbows in extension and using the scapula depressor muscles to lift the buttocks off the supporting surface (Fig. 6.5). Most persons with quadriplegia are not able to perform a wheelchair push-up in this manner and need to rely on alternative methods of weight shifting to prevent breakdown. Such methods as a lateral weight shift to each

Table 6.1
Prevalent Sites, Positions, and Possible Causes of Pressure Sores

Area	Positions Leading to Pressure	Possible Causes of Pressure
Occiput	Supine/sitting	Improperly fitting cervical orthoses
Scapula	Supine	Sliding down in bed
Vertebrae/spinous processes	Supine	Sliding down in bed
Elbow	Supine/on elbows	Excessive weightbearing, friction during mat and bed activities
Breast	Prone	Improperly fitting orthoses
Ear	Sidelying	Excessive weightbearing
Ischial tuberosity	Sitting	Worn cushion, footrests too high, poor transfer technique
Sacrum	Supine/sitting	Sliding down in bed during bed changes; kyphotic posture in wheelchair; prolonged contact with urine, feces, perspiration
Coccyx	Supine/sitting	Kyphotic position in wheelchair, poor transfer techniques
Wrist	Any position	Improperly fitting hand splints
Greater trochanter	Sidelying	Trauma during transfer, scoliosis causing increased weight shift to one hip, poor wheelchair fit
Knees	Sidelying/prone	Adductor spasms, "hammocking" of wheelchair seat
Heels	Supine/sitting	Footrests, spasms, poorly fitting shoes
Gluteal crease	Supine	Shearing forces during bed changes or transfers, moisture
Lateral malleolus	Sidelying/sitting	Trauma during transfer, poor footrest position
Medial malleolus	Sidelying	Adductor spasms
Toes	Sitting/prone	Trauma during transfer, poorly fitting shoes, poor prone positioning

side or forward over the knees are very effective pressure relief techniques (Figs. 6.6 and 6.7). If balance and upper extremity strength are poor, then a person may hook his or her arm over the back of the chair or through an adapted loop to stabilize and assist return to an upright position (Fig. 6.8). A weight shift is recommended every 15 to 20 min while in a wheelchair.

Orthotic and spinal stabilization devices, as well as clothing, should fit properly without causing excessive localized pressure or friction. Changes in the patient's activity level or weight warrant more frequent inspection of underlying tissue to ensure adequate fit of the devices. Tightly fitting clothes not only make dressing difficult but may also cause constriction of the skin and increase areas of localized pressure. Tight shoes should be eliminated for the same reasons. A person may need to purchase shoes one-half to one full size larger, owing to the changes in the vasomotor tone and an increase in dependent edema of the lower extremities following SCI.

There should not be any direct pressure on any part of the body from the wheelchair. Each patient should be measured for proper wheelchair fit. Wheelchair prescriptions take into account the weight,

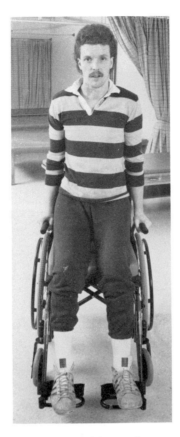

Figure 6.5. Performing a wheelchair push-up to relieve pressure.

height, activity level, and special needs of the individual, and if fitted correctly, the wheelchair should not cause excessive pressure on any area of the skin. Specific wheelchair recommendations are found in Chapter 7.

Shearing forces should be minimized during bed and mat activities. Patients should be taught to lift or "scoot," rather than drag themselves across a surface. Frictional forces should be reduced as much as possible. Using powder during sliding board transfers or wearing clothing without thick seams facilitates smoother movement. Sheets and pants should be inspected for excessive wrinkles, and linen that is roughened by laundering should be avoided.

SKIN INSPECTION

Skin inspection must be done at least twice daily, in the morning before beginning activities of daily living (ADL), such as bathing and dressing, and in the evening before sleeping. More frequent inspection is warranted if an area of the skin is susceptible to breakdown or if a new activity is initiated that results in new pressure areas or creates shearing forces. It is imperative that members of the nursing staff carry out a brief inspection at each turning schedule. Equally important is the need for the patient to carry out his or her own skin inspection.

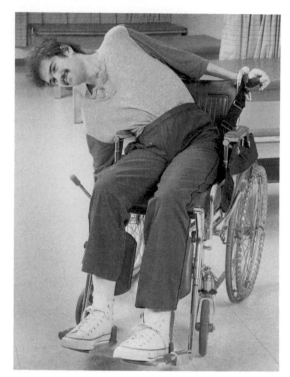

Figure 6.6.   Lateral weight shift to relieve pressure.

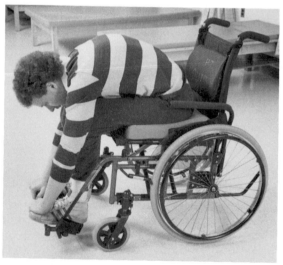

Figure 6.7.   Forward weight shift performed without stabilizing arm on wheelchair back.

Every attempt should be made to ensure that a person with a sensory loss can see and evaluate his or her own skin. A mirror can be easily adapted for the person with poor motor power in the hands (Fig. 6.9). If the person cannot hold the mirror, then he or she must be able to direct another person to hold the mirror so that both may inspect the skin.

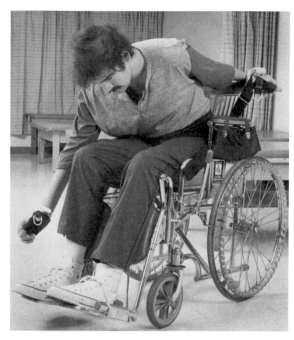

Figure 6.8. Forward weight shift performed by hooking arm over the back of wheelchair to assist return to the upright position.

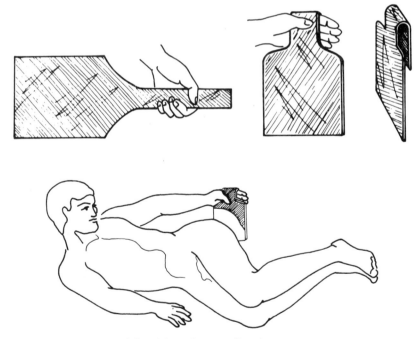

Figure 6.9. Adapted mirrors for skin inspection.

Patients must assess their skin before and immediately following ambulation using orthotic devices. Therapists must also be alert to skin breakdown and "tune in" to a quick skin assessment during range of motion (ROM) activities. It must be stressed that the primary responsibility for prevention of skin problems falls with the patient.

GENERAL HYGIENE

Personal hygiene and appearance not only enhance the psychological wellness of an individual but are also closely correlated with the presence or absence of skin problems. The bathing program should include washing with mild soap and water to avoid excessive drying and cracking of the skin. The skin should be kept clean and free from perspiration, urine, and feces. The skin must be dried thoroughly after bathing and bowel and bladder care. Special emphasis should be directed to the groin, gluteal, and toe regions because these sites are frequently predisposed to maceration. Routine lotion or alcohol rubs are avoided as the goal is for the skin to toughen naturally.

There may be increased sweating above the level of the lesion, which requires more frequent bathing and linen changes, especially for patients on bedrest. Below the level of the lesion, the skin may be excessively dry and susceptible to cracking and breakdown due to autonomic nervous system dysfunction.

Self-bathing activities for the upper extremities should be introduced when a patient is able to sit up at least 45° in bed. Lower extremity bathing begins when the patient is able to sit from 45–60° upright in bed. When bathing, patients must be cautioned not to use excessively hot water because the loss of sensation may lead to inadvertent burns.

The choice of clothing is an important consideration in the general hygiene of the patient. The type of material next to the patient's skin may either prevent or increase moisture retention while in the bed or wheelchair. Cotton clothing seems to be best for absorption and dissipation of moisture, whereas nylon and plastic materials tend to hold perspiration. Additional information on hygiene of the person with SCI is presented in Chapter 7.

NUTRITION

There are numerous reasons why a person with a SCI acquires a state of negative caloric and protein balance. In addition to loss of appetite immediately following injury, the individual has sustained significant trauma that places a large demand on the body's energy resources for recovery and healing. Proper nutrition is not only an important factor in maintaining the vitality of intact tissue but also is imperative for tissue healing. A high-protein diet with an increased caloric intake is needed initially to replace weight loss and to prevent protein deficiency and anemia. If the patient has an open sore, the problem of protein deficiency is compounded further because there is a continual loss of protein from this pressure area.

The nutritional state of the patient is also affected by drugs, alcohol, nicotine, and caffeine. Nicotine and caffeine cause vasoconstriction, which leads to a decrease in oxygenation and nourishment to the tissues. This reduction in tissue nourishment is a significant factor of concern in wound care and healing. Studies in the use of nicotine have demonstrated that patients with more pack-years of smoking habit have a higher incidence of and more extensive pressure sores than their counterparts who do not smoke.

ANTICIPATING POTENTIAL HAZARDS

The person who has a sensory loss to any part of the body must anticipate potential hazards to the skin and take precautions to prevent problems before they occur. Two of the most common hazards are the effect of external temperature changes on the skin and a change in the mental "alertness" of the person with SCI.

A variety of possibilities occurring with environmental temperature changes may result in skin breakdown. Prolonged exposure to the sun may result in severe burns. The person with sensory loss must be aware that burns not only occur from direct exposure to the sun but also from the sun's reflection off the water or sand.

The temperature of bath water must be carefully regulated to avoid burning insensitive areas. Temperature gauges should be used if there are problems with consistent temperature regulation.

Contact of the limbs with radiators, hot water pipes, car heaters, and metal may cause severe burns. Burns, however, are not the only consequence of temperature changes. Prolonged exposure to cold can cause frostbite of the fingers and toes, and special precautions need to be taken when engaging in any outdoor activity in freezing temperatures.

A change in an individual's cognitive level may lead to unsuspecting problems. The person with SCI is particularly susceptible to skin breakdown after excessive alcohol consumption. Pressure-relief techniques are either neglected or forgotten, and an individual may often remain in one position for a prolonged period of time. A change in medication may also bring about changes in cognition that lead to drowsiness and lethargy. An individual is not only "unalerted" to the need for changes in position but is also frequently unable to assist with these changes. Clinicians should also be alert to the patient's response to changes in medication and take appropriate actions to remedy any problems that may occur.

DEVICES TO ASSIST WITH PRESSURE REDUCTION

In an effort to reduce the incidence of pressure sores, numerous mattresses, special beds, wheelchair cushions, and other support systems have been developed that are claimed to prevent pressure necrosis. Although air, gel, water, and foam mattresses and cushions may be comfortable for the patient, the patient and practitioner must be cautioned about feeling "safe" when using these devices. **There is no substitute for pressure relief in the prevention of pressure sores!** With the exception of the Clinitron bed that sacrifices the mobility of the patient, no commercially available mechanical bed, cushion, or supporting device totally prevents skin breakdown. If they accomplish anything, these devices may afford an individual a few extra minutes on an area of the body before pressure causes occlusion of capillary flow. Too, some of the mechanical beds may reduce the need for physical strength or additional personnel in turning or caring for the patient. But the only answer in prevention is removal of the pressure.

This does not imply that there are not advantages to using a mattress or cushion. These devices can assist minimally with pressure relief, in addition to helping the patient's positioning, comfort, support, and posture. Some very fine cushions that assist with pressure relief are available on the market and are especially designed for the person in a wheelchair with a sensory loss. However, it is important to remember and to emphasize to the patient that the cushion cannot replace meticulous skin care and inspection.

The following criteria should be considered when selecting a device for assisting pressure relief: (a) cost of the mattress or cushion, (b) skin temperature changes occurring at the interface between patient and device, (c) pressure relief afforded by the device, and (d) effects of the mattress or cushion on mobility and transfer activities, positioning, ease of cleaning, and patient comfort. Most of the research regarding these criteria has been done on wheelchair cushions, although it may apply to mattresses of similar construction as well.

Cost may be an important consideration when selecting a permanent device for the patient, and the patient's method of payment may dictate the selection of the cushion or mattress. Cushion prices range from approximately $40 for a simple foam cushion to over $300 for a more sophisticated air-filled bladder or air/gel combination cushion. The prices are at least doubled for mattresses of the same materials. Each cushion manufacturer claims that its cushion is the most effective in relieving pressure under the ischial tuberosities; in fact, some cushions have been shown by measurement with pressure transducers under the bony landmarks to approach capillary pressures at the bone/cushion interface. At the present time, *no cushion can reduce the pressure under bony areas so that it is less than capillary pressure.*

Cushions and mattresses often increase local skin temperature, which causes an additional rise in tissue metabolism and greater oxygen demands to the area. Rubber, plastic, and gel materials are known to cause increases of temperature at their interface with the skin. The significance of increased oxygen demands in denervated tissues has been previously addressed.

The weight of a cushion may affect the demands on a patient in terms of wheelchair propulsion, endurance, and transfers. The gel cushion is heavier (up to 25 pounds) than the foam or air-filled cushion and may add to the difficulty in propelling a wheelchair for long distances or lifting a wheelchair up and down stairs whether by the patient or someone who is assisting the patient. And of course the cushion must be removed from the wheelchair for transfers in and out of the car.

In addition to trying to minimize the pressure under bony areas by the use of cushion and mattresses, cut-out boards have been custom designed to fit under a cushion in a wheelchair to provide additional relief of pressure under the ischial tuberosities. The design of a cut-out board allows a greater proportion of a person's body weight to be carried on the thighs and lateral areas of the buttocks, rather than on the ischial tuberosities and sacrum (Fig. 6.10)

This simple U-shaped board, constructed of 1/2 to 5/8-inch thick plywood, is custom cut to fit each patient and patient's wheelchair. If the cut is too narrow, the edges of the board pass directly under the

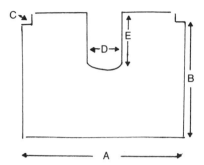

1. Begin with plywood board ½–⅝ inch thick.

2. Cut board to width (*A*) and depth (*B*) of wheelchair.

3. Notch edges (*C*) for better fit in wheelchair.

4. Measurement (D) taken with patient sidelying with hips and knees flexed. Measure distance between the ischial tuberosities and add 1 ½ to 2 inches.

5. Measurement (E) taken with the patient sitting in the wheelchair. Measure distance from the sacrum to the clearance of the perineum.

6. Cut-out opens posteriorly.

Figure 6.10.   Fabricating a cut-out board.

ischial prominences, increasing the compression and shearing forces. If the cut-out is too wide, the desired alternative weightbearing areas are reduced. The outer dimensions of the board are designed to permit easy removal of the wheelchair arms. The use of the cut-out board decreases pressure under the ischial tuberosities approximately 10–15 mm Hg. Although this is a very insignificant amount of pressure reduction, there are other advantages to using the board: The sitting posture is improved, patients' complaints of back discomfort are frequently reduced, "hammocking" of the wheelchair seat is prevented, and adductor spasticity of the lower limbs tends to be reduced. Recommended measurements for the cut-out board are shown in Figure 6.10.

The mattress or cushion may facilitate or inhibit a patient's mobility, particularly in transfer activities. Smooth surfaces offer less resistance to sliding and make board placement easier, if one is used during transfers. If an air-filled bladder-type cushion is preferred for patient use, a cushion cover should be added to facilitate transfers.

The size of a cushion may affect the back and seat heights of the wheelchair. A thick cushion raises a patient's center of gravity, which may cause an imbalance in sitting. When a cushion is fitted for a patient, the foot pedals of the wheelchair should also be adjusted. If the knees are too low in relationship to the hips, more pressure will fall on the distal thighs. If the knees are too high, more pressure will fall on the ischial tuberosities and sacrum. Softer cushions or cushions with prefabricated cut-outs may cause a "sinking effect" of the buttocks into the cut-out area and create difficulty for patients when transferring out of the wheelchair for mat or ambulation activities.

Cloth-covered foam cushions and mattresses tend to absorb moisture and are difficult to clean when incontinence and excess perspiration occur. This may prove to be an inconvenience for the patient if another cushion is not available for use during cleaning of the soiled cushion. More than one cushion or mattress cover is recommended for devices that are moisture-absorbent.

A final consideration in selecting a cushion should be the patient's comfort in using the cushion or mattress. If there is a lack of sensation, comfort may be determined by the way in which the device affects the balance, support, and positioning of the person. Additional information on cushions is found in Chapter 7.

Wound Management

Management of the pressure sore requires implementation of the same measures recommended for prevention: relief of pressure and proper hygiene. A pressure sore will not heal if there is continuous pressure on the area of breakdown. Pressure relief, optimal local hygiene, proper nutrition, an adequate hemoglobin level, and normal serum protein are prerequisites to healing, with or without surgical intervention. Given the correct methods of management, combined with patient cooperation and adequate time, the majority of pressure sores will heal without surgical intervention.

The elements of wound management then are to (1) keep the wound clean and uninfected, (2) support tissue healing by relieving pressure, and (3) maintain systemic health.

TOPICAL THERAPY

Topical therapy ranges from basic cleansing with open-air wound management to mechanical and chemical debridement methods, whirlpool, hyperbaric oxygen, electrical stimulation, and, most recently, laser therapy. Depending on the clinical situation, opinions of the medical professionals regarding the optimal treatment are as varied as the choices of treatment for wound care.

A myriad of topical agents applied in local wound treatment are used for their anti-infective properties and to stimulate growth of granulation tissue. Antibiotic agents are often used in conjunction with topical preparations because all pressure sores are colonized with bacteria (usually anaerobes and gram-negative bacilli). Some of the more commonly used agents are hydrogen peroxide, benzoyl peroxide, povidone iodine, neosporin powder, Dextranomer, and collagenase ointments.

In addition to being easy and economical, the peroxides are frequently used in clinics for their basic wound-cleansing effects. Normal saline is sometimes used in combination with hydrogen peroxide in deeper wounds to minimize the "foam" produced from the oxidizing action of the hydrogen peroxide and to assist with the removal of the cleaning agent from the wound.

The antibacterial and irritant properties of povidone iodine make it a good agent for treating the nonepithelial tissue of Grades I and II pressure sores. The povidine iodine stimulates sloughing of fibrous tissue that may cover the wound and also assists in stimulation of granulation tissue.

Neosporin powder is used in conjunction with collagenase ointment to control bacterial counts as the necrotic tissue liquifies. The liquefaction of the necrotic tissue by the collagenolytic agents facilitates its removal from the wound. Both neosporin and collagenase are most often used to treat pressure sores that are at least of Grade III severity.

Dextranomer, a granular powder composed of large dextran molecules, is used in open, draining wounds that are free of necrotic tissue. The hydrophilic action of the Dextranomer molecule reduces surrounding tissue edema and removes bacteria and by-products of tissue necrosis. It seems to be highly effective in retarding the progression or formation of sinus tracts that may arise secondary to fluid accumulation.

DEBRIDEMENT

Three methods are used to debride wounds: sharp debridement, enzymatic debridement, and mechanical debridement with cleansing and dressing techniques.

Sharp debridement is debridement using scissors, forceps, and scalpel and is often used in management of Grades II, III, and IV pressure sores. Eschar and underlying necrotic tissue are best removed by sharp debridement. Care should be taken not to cause bleeding that cannot be controlled by pressure application, and special precautions are indicated when debriding sores of patients on anticoagulant therapy. If sharp debridement is difficult due to sinus tract formation where a sore may penetrate very deeply into the tissues, then enzymatic treatment is employed in conjunction with sharp debridement.

Enzymatic preparations may be fibrinolytic or collagenolytic. Treatment with enzyme preparations causes the liquefaction of necrotic tissue and facilitates its removal by sharp or mechanical debridement. As much of the eschar as possible must be removed from the wound before enzymatic debridement or the preparation will not penetrate the eschar. Enzymatic preparations are used in the treatment of Grades II, III, and IV pressure sores.

Mechanical debridement is done by local cleansing and dressing techniques. Soap and water, or hydrogen peroxide and saline, used in a 1:3 or 1:2 ratio are some of the more common agents employed in cleansing the wound. The actions of flushing the wound with a cleansing agent, wiping it with a sterile gauze sponge, and removing gauze packing along with necrotic tissue that has adhered to the wound surface serve to clean the wound mechanically. Mechanical debridement may be carried out with every dressing change, primarily in Grades III and IV pressure sores.

DRESSING TECHNIQUES

Most Grade I and some Grade II pressure sores do not require dressings. However, when a wound requires a dressing, the basic rule for dressing changes is to allow time for damp gauze to dry and adhere to the wound and not to allow the dressing to become completely saturated with wound drainage.

Dressings should be changed at least twice daily and more often if drainage soaks through the packing. If drainage does soak through the packing, the dressing should be changed and the wound cleansed and redressed. Otherwise, the wet dressing becomes a medium for bacterial growth. The addition of dry gauze to a dressing where drainage has seeped through is contraindicated as doing so only adds bulk and greater pressure over the wound site.

An all-gauze type of dry dressing may be used in coverage of Grades I and II pressure sores, and dressing changes are carried out according to the drainage of the wound. A wet-to-dry technique is used in Grades III and IV pressure sores in the presence of necrotic tissue. A gauze is dampened with normal saline, and excessive saline is squeezed out. This gauze is placed in the wound and then covered with dry gauze. The purpose of this technique is for the underlying wet gauze to dry and adhere to the surface of the necrotic tissue. When removed, the dead tissue is pulled off with the gauze.

In small wounds, "fluffs" made from gauze strips are used to pack the wound. By using fluffs, more gauze is in contact with the wound surface, which assists with the mechanical debridement of the wound during dressing changes. If a wound is large and deep, rolled gauze instead of a gauze sponge should be used to pack the wound. If the wound is large enough to require more than one length of rolled gauze, the ends of each roll should be tied together so that no gauze will be "lost"in the wound.

A general guideline to pressure sore management is presented in Table 6.2

ADDITIONAL TREATMENT MODALITIES

Wound management and preferred treatment approaches tend to be specific to certain areas of the country or even the hospital itself. What one rehabilitation team considers to work best for them may be a completely different but equally effective treatment than is used by a neighboring facility. In addition to the previously mentioned techniques, other methods of wound management include whirlpool, hyperbaric oxygen, electrical stimulation, and laser therapy.

Table 6.2
Guidelines for Pressure Sore Management[a]

Grade I

Local cleansing
Frequent measurements of the ulcer
Grade II

Local cleansing
Gauze packing if wound is draining:
   Dextranomer to absorb drainage, sharp and enzymatic debridement if wound is necrotic
Frequent measurements of the ulcer
Grade III and IV

Local cleansing
Gauze packing:
   Dextranomer to absorb drainage, sharp and enzymatic debridement of necrotic tissue
Frequent measurements of the ulcer
Referral to plastic surgeon

---
[a] All management includes a pressure relief program for patients, family members, and members of the health care team.

Whirlpool has been a conventional treatment modality for pressure sores, and its use is still employed in many facilities. However, there are drawbacks to using whirlpool treatment. The wound may become contaminated from the water or tank. Other parts of the body are put at risk when attempting to help only one area. Shearing forces may occur during transfers from chair or bed into a tank. Other parts of the body may be susceptible to breakdown if not dried thoroughly after treatment.

A better technique that serves the same purpose as the whirlpool treatment is to treat the wound by a local application of cleaning using a surgical water pick. In a similar manner to the dentist's water pick, use of the water pick allows the therapist or nurse to direct the sterile stream of water to the wound site during treatment.

Hyperbaric oxygen therapy is the use of high-pressure, pure, humidified oxygen that is applied by a portable chamber to either the entire body or to an extremity. The chamber forces 100% oxygen into superficial tissue and assists with wound healing. Hyperbaric oxygen therapy has been found to be especially helpful with persons with SCI because it can only be used in wounds that have an intact, underlying arterial supply. This treatment modality is contraindicated in wounds with pseudomonas as it forces humidified oxygen into the wound and causes proliferation of the bacteria. When used twice a day for approximately 1 hour each treatment and when effective, wound changes may be detected within a few days.

Electrical stimulation—low voltage, direct current, and high voltage pulsed galvanic stimulation—has been used successfully in treating pressure sores. During the treatment sessions the negative electrode is placed directly in the wound, and the positive electrode is placed at some point distal to it. The negative electrode is kept in the wound during the sessions, which last approximately 1 hour, until cultures of the wound show no bacterial growth. The polarity is then switched so that the positive electrode is placed in the wound for the duration of the treatment sessions and remains that way until the wound heals, growth plateaus, or wound cultures show evidence of new infection. If wound healing stops or cultures test positive again for bacterial growth, the cycle may be repeated beginning with the negative electrode.

Laser treatments have been very effective with animal models in the treatment of pressure sores. Studies have demonstrated healing of sores using the helium-neon laser in one-third of the amount of time as compared to nonlaser treated wounds. Research in the use of laser therapy for wound healing in humans is still in its early stages of investigation. The use of laser may prove to be a very effective method of promoting wound healing.

SURGICAL INTERVENTION

Unfortunately, not all pressure sores respond to conservative measures. The longer a wound remains open, the more difficult it is to close as fibrous tissue forms around the periphery of an open, avascular wound bed. The process of surgical intervention is complicated. Along with a detailed medical evaluation, management of spasticity and contractures before surgery is of paramount importance if surgical flaps or grafts are to be successful.

Contractures, especially hip or knee flexion contractures, may interfere with patient positioning postoperatively. Most cases of plastic surgery involve the trochanters, ischia, and sacrum and require that a patient remain in the prone position continuously until the graft or flap "takes." Preoperative preparation is not only directed toward reducing the contractures but also must be directed to conditioning the patient for postsurgical positioning. Spasticity has to be managed presurgically as well, as shear stresses cause the graft or flap to displace. As with nonoperative management, patient cooperation is of utmost importance if the plastic surgery is to be successful.

Complications of Pressure Sores

If arrested early in the course of skin breakdown, all pressure sores should heal with pressure relief and conservative wound management. If these measures are not followed or if a pressure sore does not respond promptly to this type of management, the health care team should be suspicious of underlying complications. Complications of pressure sores include chronic local infection with abscess formation, sepsis, osteomyelitis, and death.

Localized soft tissue infection is one of the primary causes of fever in the spinal cord injured patient during hospitalization. The infected sore may lead to sepsis and often requires treatment with systemic antibiotic therapy in addition to debridement. Abscesses are often present beneath an infected sore, and occasionally the sore will appear to "heal over."

Osteomyelitis must always be considered if there is persistent or recurrent drainage from a wound, repeated skin breakdown in an area that seems to have healed, breakdown of plastic surgery, or unexplained fever or leucocytosis. Pain, which is normally a symptom associated with osteomyelitis, is usually absent in SCI. Osteomyelitis is caused by anaerobic bacteria and gram-negative rods, and most often arises from an infected, contiguous source, such as a pressure sore. It is often difficult to diagnose without a bone biopsy because many other conditions in SCI—osteoporosis, pressure-related bone changes, trauma—present with abnormal roentgenograms and/or nuclear imaging studies. There may be an increased uptake on the Tc-99 and Ga-77 bone scans, but bone cultures are most important in establishing the diagnosis of osteomyelitis. Bone cultures determine the causative organism, which then aids in the proper selection of antimicrobial therapy. Surgery is required in the majority of patients diagnosed with osteomyelitis.

Summary

The approach to pressure sore management is complex, and the main emphasis in skin care should be targeted to *prevention*. Every member of the health care team must understand the physiologic, psychological, social, and financial implications of skin breakdown. *The most important member and director of the team is the person with the spinal cord injury.*

Suggested Readings

Allen MS: Nursing care of the spinal cord injured patient with recurrent pressure sores. *Rehab Nurs* 9:34–36, 1984.

Bedbrook G, Beer NI, McLaren RK: Preventive measures in the tertiary care of spinal cord injured people. *Paraplegia* 23:69–77, 1975.

Dong-Myung Ma, Dong Sun Chu, Davis S: Pressure relief under the ischial tuberosities and sacrum using a cut-out board. *Arch Phys Med Rehabil* 57:352–354, 1976.

Lamid S, El Ghatit AZ: Smoking, spasticity and pressure sores in spinal cord injured patients. *Am J Phys Med* 62:300–306, 1983.

Minnis RJ, Sutton RA, Duffus A, Mattison R: Underseat pressure distribution in the sitting spinal injury person. *Paraplegia* 22:297–304, 1984.

Richardson RR, Meyer PR: Prevalence and incidence of pressure sores in acute spinal cord injuries. *Paraplegia* 19:235–247, 1981.

Staas WE, LaMantia JG: Decubitus Ulcers. In Ruskin AP (ed): *Current Therapy in Physiatry*. Philadelphia, WB Saunders, 1984.

Sugarman B: Medical complications of spinal cord injury. *Q J Med* 54:3–18, 1985.

Sugarman B: Osteomyelitis in spinal cord injury. *Arch Phys Med Rehabil* 65:132–134, 1984.

Thiyagarajan C, Silver JR: Aetiology of pressure sores in patients with spinal cord injury. *Br Med J* 289:1487–1490, 1984.

Zarro VJ: Mechanisms of inflammation and repair. In Michlovitz SL (ed): *Thermal Agents In Rehabilitation*. Philadelphia, FA Davis, 1986.

Zejdlik CM: *Management of Spinal Cord Injury*. Belmont, MA, Wadsworth Health Sciences Division, 1983.

CHAPTER 7

Physical Management

DEBORAH A. NAWOCZENSKI, M.Ed., P.T.
MARGARET E. RINEHART, M.S., P.T.
PAGE DUNCANSON, B.S., O.T.R.
BARBARA E. BROWN, B.S., O.T.R.

$\mathbf{T}$he multidisciplinary physical management and rehabilitation of the patient with spinal cord injury begin at the time of injury and continue throughout the patient's life. Within the first 24 hr of arrival at the acute care hospital, the rehabilitation team should become involved in the initiation of the treatment program. Timely intervention by the rehabilitation team helps prevent complications resulting from prolonged bedrest and promotes the early and direct involvement of the patient as the primary team member in the recovery phase.

In addition to the patient, the comprehensive management team includes the physician, nurse, physical therapist, occupational therapist, respiratory therapist, speech-language pathologist, psychologist, vocational rehabilitation specialist, and social worker. Each team member plays an integral role in optimizing the functional and social capabilities of the patient.

Each team member may play a different role in achieving the outcome. Some health care providers may concentrate on strengthening the available musculature, improving the respiratory status, or training the patient for ambulation. Other team members may be concerned with activities of daily living, the need for adaptive equipment, or driving evaluation. There are professionals involved with tracheostomy care, swallowing activities, and communication skills. Some team members provide guidance and counseling in employment opportunities, sexual options, and financial resources that are available for the patient and the family.

Not only is the integration of the various professional roles vital to the successful rehabilitation program, but equally important is the early and active family participation in the patient's recovery process.

This chapter highlights the major intervention strategies in the physical management of the patient with spinal cord injury.

Evaluation of the Patient

Physical management should begin in the intensive care unit (ICU) and progress to more aggressive treatment as the patient's medical status improves. Before any treatment program is initiated, a thorough evaluation should be performed to establish baseline information. Using this information, goals can be set for the patient and future assessments can be compared to determine progress.

Patient care is a dynamic process and so evaluations should be ongoing throughout the lifetime of the individual. Goals and subsequent treatment programs should be revised according to the evaluative findings.

Some portions of the evaluation may need to be deferred until the patient is medically and orthopedically stable. There also may be evaluation parameters more appropriate for the patient with paraplegia than quadriplegia. However, an evaluation should include as many of the following parameters as possible.

PATIENT HISTORY

The past medical history, the history of the current injury, and the social history should be included in the evaluation. Knowledge of the mechanism of injury indicates to the examiner the type of stabilization procedure that may be selected for management. An awareness of the premorbid social styles of the patient is important for setting goals and programs that are consistent with the patient's previous interests. The social history should also include information regarding the family structure or support system available to the patient.

RANGE OF MOTION

Spinal stability and precautions for movement must be clarified with the orthopedic surgeon before the initiation of any range of motion (ROM) activity. An unstable spinal fracture precludes full and aggressive joint ROM near the region of injury. Stabilization devices may interfere with attaining full ROM at a joint, and any limitations should be documented in the examiner's evaluation.

MOTOR POWER

The motor level of the patient should be determined by specific muscle testing that uses both visual and palpation skills. Palpation is important because intact muscles may substitute for paralyzed muscles in producing a desired motion. In the acute phase, the patient may not be able to assume the proper manual muscle testing positions for assigning grades to the muscles because of spinal instability or immobilization devices. Therefore, the patient's position when tested should be noted and kept consistent for subsequent muscle testing procedures.

The examiner must differentiate between isolated muscle activity and spasticity. Spasticity may give an inaccurate impression of motor recovery.

SENSATION

Light touch, pain and temperature, and proprioception sensations should be tested on each limb and trunk. The American Spinal Injury Association (ASIA) has established standards for the classification of neurologic impairment; the dermatome chart for identifying sensory areas of impairment can be found in Chapter 3.

RESPIRATORY STATUS

A complete respiratory exam should include vital capacity measurements, respiratory rate, cough force, strength of the residual respiratory muscles, and the patient's breathing pattern (see Chapter 4).

MUSCLE TONE

Muscle tone should be evaluated and attention directed to abnormal tone that may cause discomfort or hinder the patient's function. The clinician should be aware that muscle tone may change during the recovery process. Flexor tone usually predominates in the early stages of recovery in upper motor neuron injuries, and extensor tone may increase approximately 6 months postinjury. Medications that the patient is receiving to minimize abnormal tone should also be noted.

REFLEXES

Deep-tendon reflexes should be tested in all limbs and the response assessed as normal, hyperreflexic, or hyporeflexic.

SKIN

The skin should be examined for signs of local hyperemia (redness) or breakdown. The initial evaluation is the best time to begin patient education in the prevention of pressure sores and pressure relief techniques. Turning schedules must be initiated at the time of admission.

PAIN

If present, the quality, severity, and location of pain should be evaluated. The examiner should be concerned if the pain changes after admission or between evaluations.

ENDURANCE

The patient may experience cardiovascular and respiratory responses to exercise or to the evaluation process itself. These responses give the examiner an indication of the patient's baseline endurance level.

MOBILITY

Mobility testing may have to be delayed until the patient is medically and orthopedically stable. When possible, functional ability should be assessed in regard to bed mobility, transfers, static and dynamic balance, wheelchair activities, and ambulation.

BOWEL AND BLADDER MANAGEMENT

Awareness of the patient's bowel and bladder routine is important for coordinating therapy schedules and nursing management of the bowel and bladder program. The location of the legbag should be noted before ROM activities are initiated.

BEHAVIOR

The patient's behavior, responses, and reactions to the injury should be observed, along with any changes in behavior that may be detected by the health professional.

ACTIVITIES OF DAILY LIVING

When appropriate, activities of daily living (ADL), including feeding, hygiene, and dressing skills, should be assessed, noting the self-help devices that may assist the patient with any activity.

SOCIAL SITUATION

From the social standpoint, the patient's living environment, job or school situation, and the availability of financial and personal support systems should be assessed.

Mobilization of the Patient in the Intensive Care Unit

GOALS

Physical rehabilitation begins in the ICU. In this early phase of care, until the patient becomes orthopedically and medically stabilized, the goals are to (1) establish appropriate communication with the patient, particularly the ventilator-dependent patient; (2) improve and maintain a good respiratory status; (3) maintain ROM and muscle strength of remaining musculature; (4) maintain skin integrity through proper positioning and establishment of a turning schedule; (5) begin patient and family education about the goals and treatment program during this phase of management; and (6) monitor changes in the patient's status.

TREATMENT CONCEPTS IN EARLY PHASES OF CARE

Throughout all phases of care, communication and cooperation among team members are of paramount importance in maximizing the functional outcome reached by the patient. Education of peer professionals is as critical to the program's success as education of the patient. Each team member should be aware of the goals established for the patient by other members of the team so that there is consistency and carryover of the accomplishments of the treatment sessions beyond the designated treatment times.

It is important that the health care provider become familiar with the equipment and machines used in patient management, especially in the ICU. There are special beds, stabilization devices, and monitoring equipment used during the treatment program. It is possible that some of the bedside activities may trigger a monitor's alarm. The nurse and therapist who are familiar with the equipment will respond appropriately when intervention is necessary.

Respiratory Care. The respiratory program should include deep breathing exercises, postural drainage, intermittent positive pressure breathing, coughing, incentive spirometry, and strengthening of the respiratory muscles. Any deterioration of the patient's status signals an emergency situation. Guidelines for respiratory management are discussed in Chapter 4.

Positioning and Range of Motion. Proper positioning in bed is necessary to prevent skin breakdown and to maintain the extremities in positions that minimize joint contractures. Contractures can significantly limit a patient's functional ability. ROM exercises performed at least twice a day and proper positioning while in bed prevent contractures.

Special attention should be directed to preventing the common and troublesome contractures that may occur in the upper extremities in the patient with quadriplegia. Frequently, a patient assumes a posture in bed that may be described as a "coffin position." As the term implies, the patient assumes a position of shoulder flexion, adduction, and internal rotation; elbow flexion; and forearm pronation. Tightness then develops in these joint positions because the patient with a high cervical cord injury does not have the motor ability to place the arms in the opposing positions.

The patient with a cervical cord injury usually requires assistance for positioning of the upper extremities, and attention should be directed to maintain full ROM in shoulder abduction, extension, and external rotation; elbow extension; and forearm supination. Contractures of these joints interferes with functional activities that require a good range of shoulder and elbow motion, such as sitting and transfer activities (Fig. 7.1).

Full flexion and extension of the wrist, metacarpal phalangeal (MP), and intercarpal phalangeal (IP) joints must be maintained with daily ROM. One exception to the general rule of preventing contractures or tightness applies to the treatment of the finger flexor and extensor muscle tendons. Although it is important to maintain full *joint* mobility of the wrist and hand, the therapist should not overstretch the finger flexor and extensor tendons.

The reciprocal ROM of finger extension coupled with wrist flexion, and of wrist extension coupled with finger flexion, is an important concept in the care of the quadriplegic hand. Range of motion that is performed in this manner permits the desired tightness to develop in

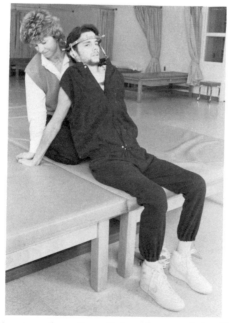

Figure 7.1. Good range of motion of the elbow and shoulder is necessary for functional activities.

the flexor and extensor tendons. Therefore, when the wrist is extended, the tightness and pull of the flexor tendons being stretched over the wrist cause the fingers to flex into the palm of the hand. This *tenodesis* action provides a functional grasp to the patient who has only the motor ability to extend (or dorsiflex) the wrist. Likewise, when the wrist is relaxed into flexion, tightness of the finger extensors being stretched over the dorsum of the wrist causes the fingers to open and the grasp to release.

At rest, the hand should be positioned with the wrist in slight extension and the fingers flexed to assist with optimal tenodesis function. Wrist splints may be used to maintain proper wrist and finger position, and the thumb should be held in opposition. The wearing time for splints should begin with a 2-hr on/off schedule and should be increased gradually if there are no signs of excessive pressure from the splints.

In the acute management of the patient with cervical spine instability or fracture, ROM exercises should be limited to 90° of shoulder flexion and abduction to avoid undue stress to the site of injury.

In the lower extremities, contractures commonly occur in the hip flexor, knee flexor, and ankle plantarflexor muscle groups. (Hip and knee flexor contractures usually occur after prolonged sitting or long-standing flexor spasticity and may not develop in the early phases of management). Emphasis should be placed on maintaining sufficient ROM in the hamstrings and gastroc-soleus muscles. The goal of unilateral straight-leg raising (hamstring stretching) is 110° in order for the patient to maintain a stable long-sitting position. This long-sitting position is necessary when the patient learns dressing techniques and when he or she must move the lower extremities in preparation for transfers and bed activities (Fig. 7.2).

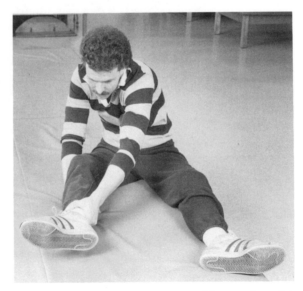

Figure 7.2.   Adequate hamstring flexibility is needed for transfer and dressing activities in the long-sitting position.

If the patient has tight hamstrings, he or she may experience difficulty in balancing in the long-sitting position and may fall backward. In attempting to get the head and trunk forward, the patient frequently stretches the back musculature. If the back becomes too flexible, the patient may suddenly "jack-knife" forward during transfers and sitting activities. The action of the trunk suddenly flexing forward is described as "telescoping" and occurs in patients who have excessive trunk mobility. Selective tightness of the back musculature is desirable to provide stability to the trunk during transfers and mat activities and to allow for maximum utilization of the upper extremity muscle power to move the buttocks and hips.

Although hip and knee flexion contractures are not common in the *early* phases of recovery, attention should still be directed to preventing these contractures. If present, they will interfere with ADL, transfers, mat and bed mobility, and if appropriate, ambulation.

The prone position is best for the prevention of hip and knee flexion contractures. The prone position may be contraindicated for the acutely injured and unstable patient, but it should be encouraged as soon as the patient is medically stable.

Ankle dorsiflexion to 90° (or neutral) is necessary for future positioning of the feet in a wheelchair. Sufficient ankle dorsiflexion is also important for the patient who may have the potential to stand and/or ambulate during later phases of recovery.

Ankle splints or high-top sneakers may assist with the prevention of contractures, and a wearing schedule of 2-hr off/on can be gradually lengthened. Boards that are positioned at the foot of the bed for the purpose of preventing foot drop are not recommended for the patient with SCI. Pressure from the board on the ball of the foot may facilitate extensor spasticity in the lower extremity. In addition, if the insensate foot is not placed correctly against the footboard, abnormal pressures may develop and cause skin breakdown.

Family members should be instructed in ROM exercises, positioning, and turning procedures and be alerted to any precautions that need to be followed during these activities. Moreover, the patient should gradually assume responsibility for his or her positioning, turning schedule, and skin inspection.

Strengthening Exercises. Until the patient is orthopedically stable, an aggressive strengthening program is contraindicated. In the ICU, active assisted exercise of the innervated muscle groups may be initiated, but should not produce any stress or stretching of the tissues around the fracture site.

When the patient is cleared for an increased activity level, the strengthening program should be augmented to include active and resistive exercises. The muscles should be selectively strengthened for carryover to functional skills.

Acute and Comprehensive Rehabilitation

The acute rehabilitation phase begins when the patient is both medically and surgically stable for mobilization out of bed. Functional skills are introduced in the acute phase of management, along with preparations for re-entry into the home and community. However, there still may be many medical complications in the acute rehabilitation phase that may interfere with the smooth progression of the patient's program. The patient should be taught to recognize potential medical complications and know proper intervention strategies that he or she may follow to avert some of the complications. These medical complications were addressed in Chapter 3.

Although the complications of SCI may continue throughout the lifetime of an individual, most complications should be resolved before the beginning of the comprehensive rehabilitation phase of care. Treatment programs that were initiated in the acute phase should intensify in accordance with increases in the patient's endurance and level of ability. In this phase of recovery, strong emphasis should be placed on patient education. Each member of the interdisciplinary team must educate the patient and family so that all aspects of care are understood.

Plans for equipment, assistive devices, and home modifications need to be finalized in preparation for discharge. Finally, physical management in the follow-up phase of care should focus on prevention of complications and health maintenance.

GOALS OF THE PROGRAM

Throughout the physical management process, goals should be continually reassessed and modified according to the patient's progress. The goals in the acute and comprehensive phases of care incorporate those previously outlined for the patient in the ICU. In addition, they include to (1) increase endurance, strength, and balance; (2) progressively mobilize the patient from bed, to wheelchair, to mat, and to ambulation activities, if appropriate; (3)channel motor activity into functional skills; and (4) plan for discharge.

Treatment Approaches

SPINAL ORTHOSES

The functions of a spinal orthosis are to support, immobilize, and protect the spine. Orthoses are primarily selected according to their effectiveness in immobilization. The control afforded by an orthosis may vary from minimum or least effective control of movement to intermediate control, to most effective control of movement. The rehabilitation team should be aware of the functions, limitations, and precautions associated with the prescribed orthosis. Treatment programs may need to be modified as dictated by the limitations imposed by the device.

CERVICAL ORTHOSES

Halo Orthosis. The halo device is one of the most effective orthoses for limiting movement in the cervical spine. The patient may have some difficulty performing functional activities, however, when wearing this device. The added weight and the location of the orthosis result in a higher-than-normal center of gravity, which causes the patient to be top-heavy and may interfere with his or her balance during transfers and sitting activities. Most of the patients adjust to the higher balance point, but will have to relearn a skill when the orthosis is removed.

The design of the vest prevents full shoulder flexion, extension, and abduction. The inferior border of the vest may cause discomfort because of its position on the abdomen. To make the patient more comfortable while supine, additional pillows can be propped under the patient's back.

The pins should not cause discomfort after the first 48 hr following application. However, if the pins are not routinely tightened, they may loosen and cause pain, discomfort, and infecton. Use of a disinfectant around the pin sites on a daily basis ensures that the pins are observed regularly for signs of loosening.

The halo vest should be examined for areas of tightness and trimmed at points of excessive skin friction caused by repetitive movements of the upper extremities. If the vest is designed to permit observation of the underlying skin, the scapula, ribs, acromion process, and spinous processes should be carefully inspected. The patient who has a sensory loss is not able to discern areas of pressure under the vest. The therapist and nurse should observe for local changes, such as increased warmth and inflammation in adjacent regions of the skin, and systemic changes, such as fever and malaise, which may indicate a pressure sore formation.

The liner between the skin and the vest should be kept dry to prevent maceration and skin breakdown and should be changed monthly. Powder should not be used on the skin under the vest as it may contribute to pressure areas.

SOMI (Sterno-Occipital-Mandibular-Immobilizer). The SOMI orthosis povides intermediate control of movement in the cervical spine. Both occipital and mandibular components anchor from the anterior (sternal) attachment and can be applied while the patient is supine.

Adjustments may be needed when the patient changes from a supine to a sitting position. The mandibular component should be moved superiorly to maintain alignment of the orthosis. Likewise, when the patient returns to a supine position, the mandibular component should be moved inferiorly. If it is not positioned correctly, the mandibular piece may press against the throat and cause the patient to experience difficulty with swallowing.

The skin should be examined for areas of increased pressure. Pillows should not be placed under the patient's head in the supine position, but may be used for support when the patient is in the sidelying position.

Philadelphia Collar. The Philadelphia collar is a two-piece lightweight polyethylene foam collar that provides intermediate-to-minimal control of movement. Occasionally the collar causes irritation and perspiration buildup. Male patients often grow a beard to minimize the rubbing, or both male and female patients may wear a silk scarf under the collar.

On occasion, tightness of the collar anteriorly may interfere with the patient's swallowing function. An alternative method of stabilization may be appropriate if this restriction persists.

THORACOLUMBAR ORTHOSES

Clam Shell or Molded Body Jacket. The body jacket, a two-piece polypropylene-molded shell, provides intermediate to most effective control of movement. The inferior border of the jacket may limit the patient's ability to sit at 90° (trunk-hip angle) in the wheelchair or in the long-sitting position.

The jacket may need to be trimmed in the areas where muscle hypertrophy from strength training programs has occurred. Commonly, the pectoralis and latissimus muscles become quite developed in the patient with paraplegia and tend to rub along the margins of the body jacket if it is not trimmed.

The shell can be removed while the patient is prone or supine to examine the skin at the bony areas of contact with the brace. The patient should also wear a cotton T-shirt under the jacket to minimize perspiration effects.

Knight-Taylor and Jewett Hyperextension Orthoses. Both orthoses give intermediate control of movement and primarily restrict forward bending. The Jewett brace is less cumbersome and encompassing than the Knight-Taylor, but the location of the anterior/inferior support pad at the superior pubis level may interfere with transfers and long-sitting activities that require sitting to at least 90°. If either orthosis does not fit properly, it will slide up on the patient's trunk and cause loss of adequate stabilization.

Both orthoses allow for visual inspection of the underlying skin for signs of pressure concentration.

MOBILIZATION FROM BED TO WHEELCHAIR

In preparation for out-of-bed and wheelchair activities, the head of the bed should be progressively elevated to increase the patient's tolerance of an upright position. The patient should be observed for any signs of respiratory or cardiac distress and *postural hypotension.* As previously recommended, abdominal binders may be used to support the diaphragm in a better functional position and to minimize the effects of postural hypotension. Antiembolic stockings or ace-wraps on both lower limbs also help decrease hypotensive effects.

When the patient can tolerate a 60° elevation in bed for approximately 1 hr, he or she is ready for transfer to a reclining wheelchair with elevating legrests. The reclining back of the chair should be elevated in 5–10° increments, according to the patient's tolerance as measured by blood pressure monitoring. Legrests should also be gradually lowered. The length of time in the wheelchair should be increased until the patient is able to tolerate being out of bed throughout the entire day.

DEVELOPMENT OF WHEELCHAIR SKILLS

Weight Shifting Techniques.   Weight shifts should be done every 20–30 min while the patient is in the wheelchair. Most patients do not have the sensory feedback to "cue" them at a subconscious level when it is time to shift weight off an area. Therefore, patients need frequent reminders in the early phases of treatment until, it is hoped, pressure relief techniques become automatic to them.

If the patient is dependent for wheelchair weight shifting, the techniques can be done by another person in the following manner: (1) the chair can be tilted backward; (2) the patient in a reclining wheelchair can be alternately rolled to each side for a few minutes every 30 min; and (3) the armrest of the chair can be removed, and the patient can be shifted to his or her side to rest on a mat table or bed for a few minutes.

Pressure relief techniques for the patient who has adequate balance and strength to perform the weight shift independently were discussed in Chapter 6. Patients may alternately shift their trunk laterally or forward after stabilizing their arm around the push-handle of the chair, or those who have functional tricep strength may perform a wheelchair push-up by placing their arms on the wheel or armrest and locking them in extension before lifting the buttocks off the seat.

The push-up weight shift technique may cause the patient's trunk to suddenly flex forward as the center of gravity shifts cranially and further anteriorly during this technique. Therefore, good sitting balance and trunk control are prerequisites for the patient who performs the push-up for weight shifting.

The patient who has adequate upper extremity strength and some trunk control may be able to "pop" and maintain a wheelie for the purpose of weight shifting. The change of position results in pressure shift off the normal weightbearing areas.

Cushions, seatboards, and other adaptive seating devices can assist with posture maintenance and weight distribution, but there are no substitutes for timely pressure-relief techniques.

Propelling the Wheelchair.   The forward push of wheelchair propulsion is accomplished through the action of the shoulder flexors, adductors, and external rotators. Propelling a wheelchair backward requires the use of shoulder extensors, adductors, and internal rotators. Additional power can be added to the push by the actions of trunk flexion and extension.

Some wheelchair adaptations may be necessary for the patient who has weak upper extremities and/or poor hand function. Plastic-coated hand-rims or rubber tubing laced around the rims may improve the efficiency of the push by providing for better friction between the pushing hand and the wheel rim. Projections (lugs), either vertical, oblique, or horizontal, are often added to wheelchair rims to gain additional propulsion power. However, projections that are not vertical increase the overall width of the chair and may cause problems for the patient who has to negotiate the chair through narrow doorways. The use of projections also encourages more bicep muscle activity for propulsion. The potential exists for this muscle to develop a contracture.

The patient may also wear wrist splints, suede hand cuffs, or gloves (similar to biking gloves) to improve efficiency in propelling the chair. The patient who has sufficient hand function usually does not require any adaptations to assist with propulsion. All patients, however, need to learn how to maneuver the chair in all environments and on all terrains.

Electric Wheelchair Propulsion.   An electric wheelchair may be prescribed for the patient who has sustained a high cervical cord injury or whose life-style demands quicker mobility and greater energy conservation, such as a college life-style.

There are a variety of options to consider when selecting an electric wheelchair. These options include (a) the wheelchair controls, either chin and/or tongue control, sip-and-puff breath control, or hand control; (2) reclining systems that allow the patient to change positions and shift weight; (3) ventilator adaptations to accommodate portable ventilator equipment; and (4) accessories to assist with head, trunk, and extremity support during operation.

It is important for the patient to become familiar with the wheelchair's features and operation. The patient should assume responsibility for battery maintenance and charging. Most wheelchairs require overnight battery charging to ensure continous operation throughout the day.

Operating an electric wheelchair requires practice in starting, stopping, turning, and negotiating ramps and obstacles. The goal is for propulsion to be smooth and safe.

MANAGEMENT OF THE WHEELCHAIR COMPONENTS

For the patient who is immobilized in an orthosis, management of the wheelchair may be difficult. However, the patient should attempt to assist with management of the brakes, armrests, and legrests as much as possible. The patient should be knowledgeable in all aspects of maintenance and management of the wheelchair. In this way, the dependent patient is at the very least able to instruct others who may assist with managing the chair.

Brake Management.   *Push-to-lock toggle brakes* are the easiest brakes to operate. Locking and unlocking of the wheelchair brakes should not pose a problem for the patient who has intact wrist extensors. Brake extensions may be considered for the patient who has weak or absent wrist extensors or who has difficulty reaching and locking the brakes. Problems may be encountered during transfers unless the brake extensions are removed. As the patient's balance and strength improve, managing the brakes without the extension is a realistic goal.

Armrest Management.   Removing the armrests of the wheelchair is facilitated with a *quad release button:* a flat lever that pushes the pin out of the hole that locks the armrest into the chair frame.

When lifting the armrests off the chair, the patient must lift from the center of the armrest panel or the front or back strut will jam.

After removing the armrest in preparation for transfer, the patient should place the armrest in a position where it can be easily retrieved and reattached to the chair (preferably on the push-handle or rear armrest holder).

Legrest/Footrest Management. Legrest management is more difficult than brake and armrest management. Some legrests detach and reattach from the front of the chair and may be easier to manage for the patient with quadriplegia. Other legrests swing to the side before removal and reattachment.

The main difficulty a patient may encounter is trying to locate the lever that releases the pedal. The *cam release mechanism* is recommended for the patient with quadriplegia because it is easier to manipulate than pin locks on a legrest. The patient should develop his or her own technique in hitting or pulling the lever to release the footpedal (Figs. 7.3 and 7.4).

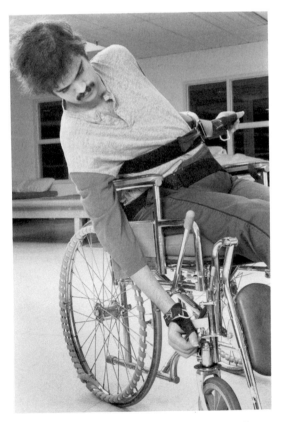

Figure 7.3. The wheelchair has several adaptations to assist the person with weak upper extremities. Rubber tubing has been placed on the wheel rims to improve propulsion ability. Suede hand mitts help provide better friction for pushing. Brake extensions aid locking and unlocking. Extensions have also been added to armrest and legrest levers.

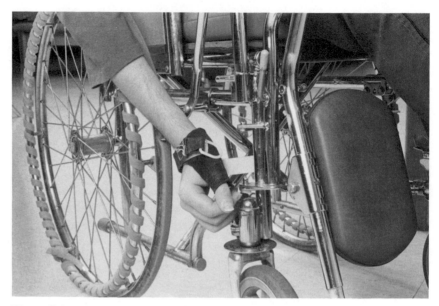

Figure 7.4.   The cam release mechanism on the legrest, with or without an extension, is often easier to manipulate than pin locks. To release the mechanism, a person can use the thenar eminence, fingers, or dorsum of the hand.

ADVANCED WHEELCHAIR SKILLS

The patient should be instructed in managing the wheelchair on different terrains. More difficult terrains require greater strength and body momentum and a good combination of timing and coordination. If independence is an unrealistic goal on various terrains, the patient should still know how to manage or be able to instruct another person how to manage the chair.

Wheelies.   The wheelie is often considered the cornerstone of advanced wheelchair activities. Wheelies permit the person to negotiate curbs and rough terrain, such as gravel or small hills.

There are a few ways to teach a patient how to assume and maintain a wheelie position. Initially, the patient should be placed in a wheelie position by the therapist to acquire a sense of the balance point in this position. When the patient is comfortable in this position, he or she should be instructed to "pop" a wheelie. Some patients find it easier to pop a wheelie by using a three-step method: (1) Without removing the hands off the wheels, the patint wheels forward; (2) then backward; and (3) quickly forward again with enough impetus to lift the front castors off the floor (Fig. 7.5). The patient should learn to readjust his or her hand positions on the wheel to maintain the balance point. The patient should be guarded closely while learning this skill, but not hindered in his or her movement.

After the patient can assume and maintain a wheelie, he or she should learn to move forward, backward, and to turn while holding the wheelie position.

Ramps and Curbs.   Ramps may be descended in a wheelie position. However, the safest method for the patient to descend a ramp is

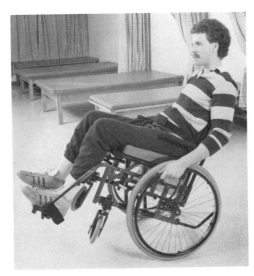

Figure 7.5. Finding the balance point is a prerequisite to popping and maintaining a wheelie position.

backward. The patient must remember to lean forward into the ramp to prevent the chair from tipping backward. Ascending ramps also require the patient to lean forward while propelling the chair up the ramp (Fig. 7.6). *Grade-aids*, a device that retards the backward movement of the wheels when the patient has to readjust his or her hand position, may facilitate the patient's ascent on steep ramps.

Curbs present a greater challenge to the patient. The patient should be able to climb a 2-inch curb by popping the front castors onto the curb and then leaning the trunk forward while pulling the rear wheels up. The patient must approach curbs that are higher than 4–5 inches in a wheelie position. Once the front castors are on the curb, the technique of pulling the rear wheels up onto the curb is the same as maneuvering the 2-inch curb. Successful negotiation of higher curbs demands better coordination and timing.

The easiest method of descending the curb is to wheel backward. The patient should back to the edge of the curb and control the rear wheels while slowly lowering the chair. At the same time, the patient should lean forward over the knees to prevent the chair from tipping backward. The patient must remember to lower the rear wheels off the curb evenly. After the rear wheels are down the curb, the patient can pivot the front castors off the curb or pop a wheelie and turn the chair.

Some patients prefer to descend a curb forward while maintaining a wheelie position. This method is more difficult as the patient must remember to lower the front castors as soon as the rear wheels contact the ground. Otherwise, the chair may tip backward (Fig. 7.7).

Stairs.   When ascending stairs in a wheelchair, the wheelchair must be backed up the steps. Unless the patient has excellent upper body strength, and has a lightweight wheelchair, ascending stairs usually requires the assistance of two people. The patient may assist

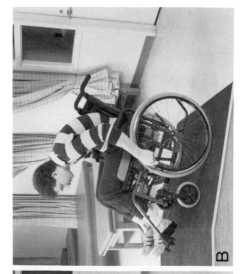

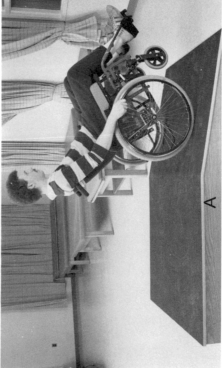

Figure 7.6. *A*, A person with good wheelchair mobility skills may be able to descend a ramp in a wheelie position. *B*, The safest method to descend a ramp is backward. The person must remember to lean forward while controlling the rear wheels. Ascending a ramp is performed in a similar manner.

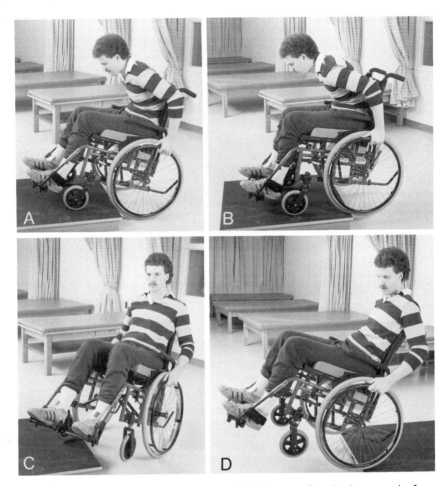

Figure 7.7. *A* and *B*, A person ascends a curb by "popping" a wheelie to get the front castors onto the curb, then pulls the rear wheels up. Timing and good upper extremity strength are important for this activity. *C*, Descending a curb may be performed by lowering the rear wheels evenly off the curb and completing the activity by spinning the chair to clear the front castors. *D*, A person may descend the curb forward in a controlled wheelie position.

with this activity by controlling or holding the rear wheels while the persons pulling the chair to the next higher step reposition their feet.

When descending stairs, the approach may be forward or backward. Again, the patient may attempt to assist the descent by controlling the wheels while the persons assisting reposition their feet.

Occasionally, the patient is able to descend stairs using one or two railings. While holding onto the railings, the patient must control the backward descent by lowering the rear wheels evenly off one step at a time. It is important for the person to lean forward while controlling the descent.

Falling. It is inevitable that at some time the patient will fall out of the chair. The patient should be prepared for this event by learning how to prevent injury when falling out of the wheelchair and how to get back into the chair.

As soon as patients feel their chair starting to tip backward beyond the balance point, they should quickly tuck their chin, turn their head, and use their arms to block their knees from hitting their face (Fig. 7.8). The push-handles of the chair usually absorb the initial impact. Once the chair is on the ground, the patients who have functional upper body strength can slide out the back of the chair, tip it upright, and transfer back into the chair from the floor.

Patients who have very good upper body strength and coordination may opt to remain in the chair and use their arms to push themselves and the chair to an upright position. Some patients "walk" one arm along the side of the chair while flexing the trunk forward to bring the front castors down to the floor (Fig. 7.9).

TRANSFER TRAINING

All activities, whether transfers, bed mobility, ADL, or ambulation, should be directed toward some functional outcome. Most skills may be broken down into their component parts, which eventually lead up to the expected outcome. The term "lead up" implies a component or part of an activity, such as balance, flexibility, or strength, that contributes to the successful acquisition of the skill. Lead-up activities allow the patient to achieve some measure of success at each treatment session while still focusing on the desired goal.

Attainment of a skill requires a problem-solving approach from both the patient and therapist. The more approaches or styles that a patient develops, the more independent that person will be. The person should develop techniques that are appropriate for his or her age, body type, flexibility, strength, life-style, and home/work environments. Experimentation, patience, and persistence are keys to a successful outcome.

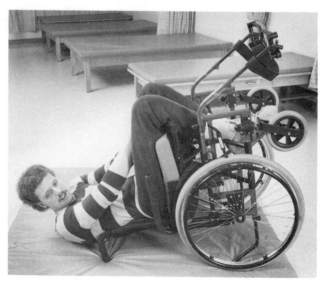

Figure 7.8.   When falling backward, a person must learn to tuck his chin quickly, turn his head, and block his knees with his hands so they do not hit the face.

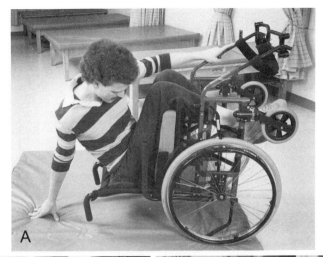

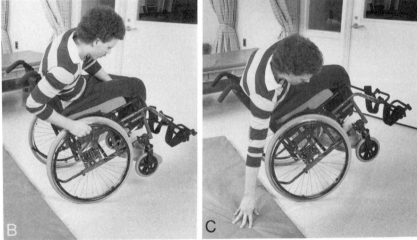

Figure 7.9. A person with excellent upper body strength may be able to right the wheelchair without getting out of the chair.

Transfer training is an important aspect of treatment for the person with a SCI. Initially, the patient may be completely dependent in transfers. High-level quadriplegic patients will remain dependent in transfers throughout their lifetime. However, the person with paraplegia should become independent in transfers to a bed, commode, car, tub, sofa, or the floor and usually will not require adaptive equipment for the activity.

Many approaches can be used to accomplish the same goal. One approach for each type of transfer is presented below as a guideline for the clinician.

Two-Person Lift. A two-person lift may be needed to transfer the patient with a high-level SCI. Care must be taken not to scrape the patient's buttocks across the wheel during the transfer. The persons assisting with the transfer must be acutely aware of proper body mechanics during the lift. Figure 7.10 illustrates the two-person lift.

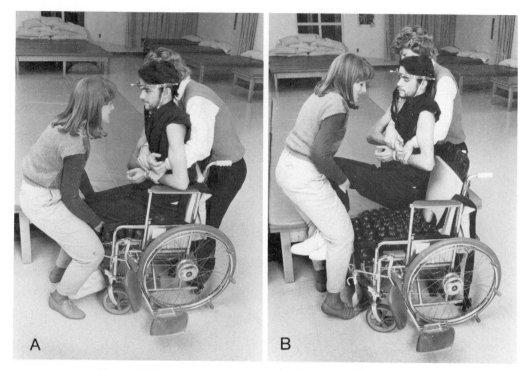

Figure 7.10. Care must be taken so that the patient's buttocks clear the wheel during the two-person lift. Good body mechanics are equally important for the persons assisting with this type of transfer.

Stand-Pivot Transfer (Therapist Assist). Frequently, a therapist may want to concentrate on a particular mat or bed activity during the treatment session and does not want the patient to be fatigued by the transfer. The stand-pivot transfer (SPT) technique requires one person who uses good body mechanics and leverage principles to carry out the transfer. The techniques of the transfer are demonstrated in Figure 7.11.

Airlift. An airlift technique is sometimes used in preference to a SPT or when a patient has severe extensor spasticity that may increase when pressure is applied to the plantar surface of the foot, as in standing. The patient is lifted through the air and does not bear any weight on the extremities during the transfer. Figure 7.12 depicts the airlift technique.

Sliding Board Transfer. Sliding boards bridge the gap between transferring surfaces. Various adaptations on a sliding board allow it to be positioned easier for patients with limited grasp (Fig. 7.13). There are also boards available with a metal bar spring attached to the underside of the board that can be placed in the wheelchair's armrest holder and pivoted under the person for the transfer (Fig. 7.14).

Body proportions play a factor in the amount of lift a patient can achieve while transferring. Longer arms locked in extension facilitate a higher lift so that the buttocks do not drag during the transfer. Figure 7.15 illustrates the sliding board transfer.

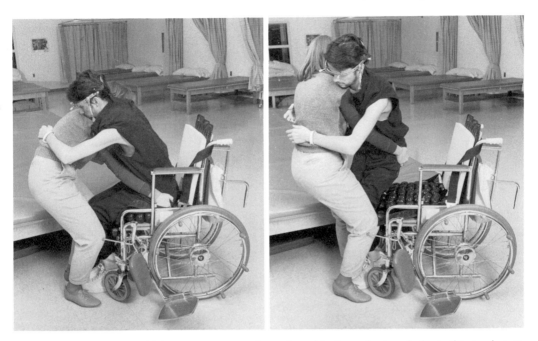

Figure 7.11. Leverage principles and good body mechanisms facilitate this stand-pivot transfer. The patient may assist with this transfer by holding his or her arms around the person who is transferring.

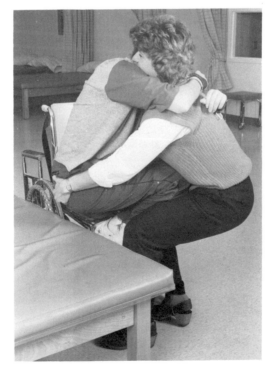

Figure 7.12. In the airlift transfer, the patient's flexed legs rest on or between the therapist's thighs. The patient can be "rocked" out of the chair and lifted onto the bed or mat. All the weight is carried through the therapist's legs and not the back.

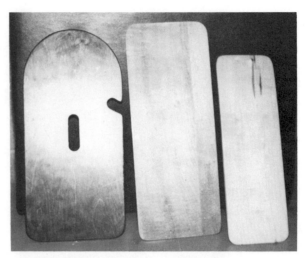

Figure 7.13.   Transfer (sliding) boards are available in all shapes and sizes. Adaptations should be left to therapist and patient innovativeness.

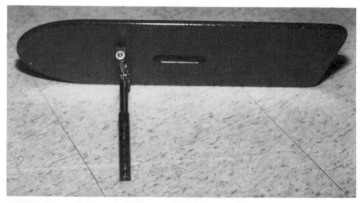

Figure 7.14.   The transfer (sliding) board is adapted with a metal bar spring attached to the board. The bar can be placed in the wheelchair armrest holder.

Stand-Pivot Transfer (Patient Performs Independently).   If a person has good trunk control in a short sitting position, and is able to perform a wheelchair push-up, he or she may be able to perform a stand-pivot transfer without therapist assistance or use of a sliding board. The person must remember to lift the buttocks, rather than drag across the wheels during the transfer (Fig. 7.16A, 7.16B).

Lateral and Forward Transfers.   The patient who has good upper extremity strength and balance in the long-sitting position, as well as good hamstring flexibility, may perform a lateral or forward transfer onto the mat or bed.

In the lateral transfer, the patient places the lower extremities onto the mat and then performs a long-sitting push-up onto the mat surface. The patient can also transfer forward out of the chair after placing the legs onto the mat and can then perform a series of long-sitting push-ups until the transfer is completed. The sequence is

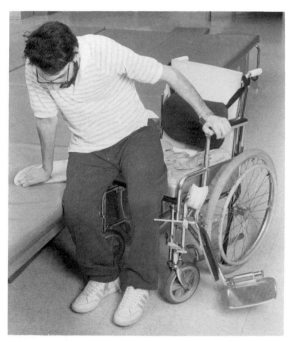

Figure 7.15. A person performing a sliding board transfer must lift or "scoot" the buttocks across the board. Tenodesis should be maintained for any upper extremity weightbearing activity.

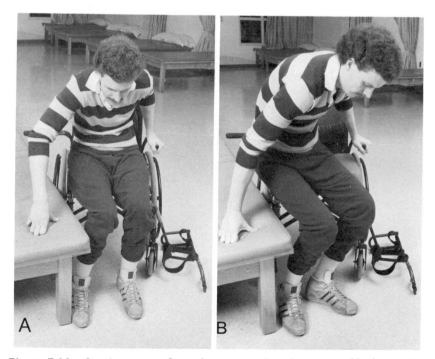

Figure 7.16. Stand-pivot transfer without using a board requires stable short-sitting balance and good upper extremity strength. By quickly twisting/moving the head and shoulders opposite to the direction of desired hip movement, a person can gain additional momentum for the transfer.

reversed when returning to the wheelchair. Figure 7.17 shows the lateral and forward transfer techniques.

In all techniques, the manner in which the wheelchair is positioned adjacent to the transferring surface is important for an effective transfer. A 45° angle to the mat reduces the width between the transferring surfaces and places the rear wheel of the chair away from the area of transfer. This angle between the chair and transferring surface is an optimal position for most transfers.

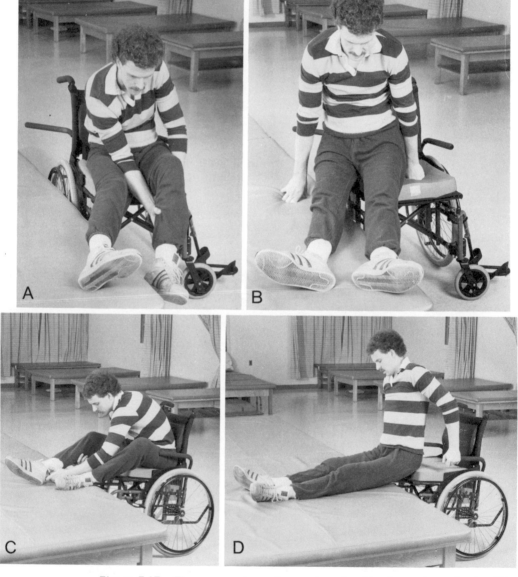

Figure 7.17. The person who performs a lateral and/or forward transfer should be able to maneuver the lower extremities and do a long-sitting push-up in preparation for these transfers.

There are many variations to the previously described methods. The challenge is to be creative. There is no right way or wrong way for a patient to perform an activity. Nonetheless, there often is a "better" way.

MAT ACTIVITIES

A mat program should have functional carryover to daily activities. Lead-up exercises that incorporate a particular movement or series of movements from certain skills should be designed to enhance the patient's strength, balance, and coordination. The nature and value of an exercise program change with each phase of recovery and emphasis of management.

Mat Progression. *Rolling* is one of the first activities in the patient's mat program. This activity is necessary so that a patient can assist with positional changes in bed, and it is preparatory to more advanced skills, such as dressing.

The patient should begin the roll from a sidelying position, progress to supine with the legs crossed in the intended direction of the roll, and finally progress to supine with the legs uncrossed. The patient should use the head, scapula, upper trunk, and arms to gain sufficient momentum to complete the roll (Fig. 7.18). The patient who has recently been released from cervical immobilization is very weak in the neck musculature and will have difficulty with this technique.

The patient may progress from the roll to a prone or sidelying position. From the prone position, a patient can work to the *prone-on-elbows position*, proceeding to a long-sitting position by "walking" the forearms toward the feet, using the head against the mat, if necessary, to assist with the movement. The patient may then hook the arm around the leg(s) and attempt to pull the trunk over the legs to reach the long-sitting position. The patient is most stable in this position with arms fully extended behind the hips. Figures 7.19A through 7.19E illustrate this progression.

A patient may also attain a long-sitting position from a supine to *supine-on-elbows position*. There are a few· techniques to reach a supine-on-elbow position before progressing to long-sitting. A patient who has strong triceps may be able to push him- or herself from a supine position, to supine-on-elbows and finally extend the elbows to reach a full long-sitting position. The patient who is paraplegic should not have difficulty with this technique, but the person with quadriplegia usually needs an alternative method.

A patient may be able to assume a supine-on-elbows position by manipulating the hands under the hips or into the pants pocket. With the hands as the distal stabilization point, the patient can use reverse action of the wrist extensors and/or biceps to pull the trunk midway into the position. To complete the activity, the patient must shift his or her weight from side to side and alternately reposition the elbows until they are under the shoulders (Fig. 7.20).

From the supine-on-elbows position, a patient may shift his or her weight to one elbow and fling one arm at a time behind the back, locking the elbow in extension. By shifting the trunk weight over the

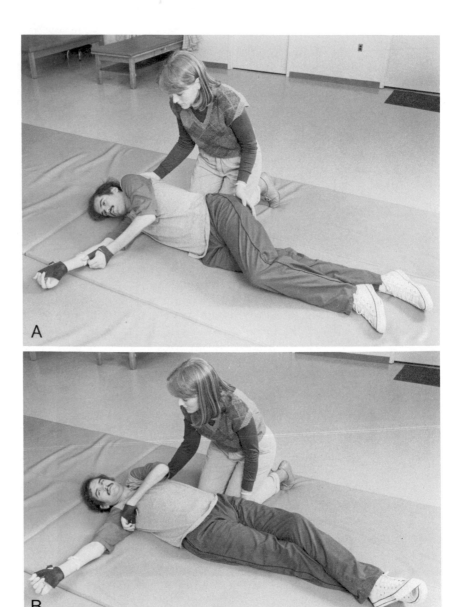

Figure 7.18. Rolling may be initiated from the sidelying or supine positions. When able, the patient should use head and arm movements to gain momentum for the roll.

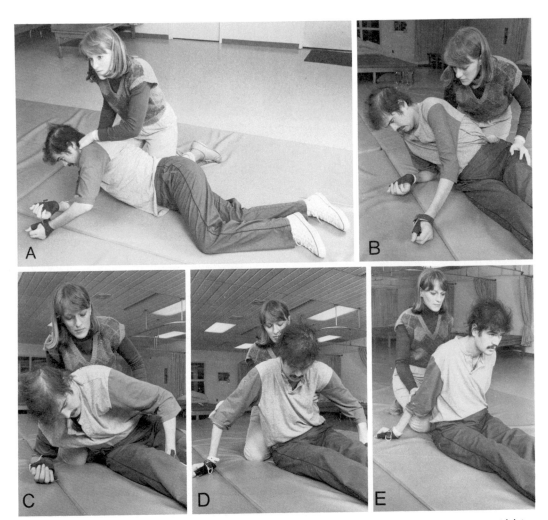

Figure 7.19. The progression to long-sitting may begin from the prone or sidelying position. The combination of weight shifting and "walking" the elbows toward the feet enables the person to hook one arm around the leg to pull him- or herself to a long-sitting position.

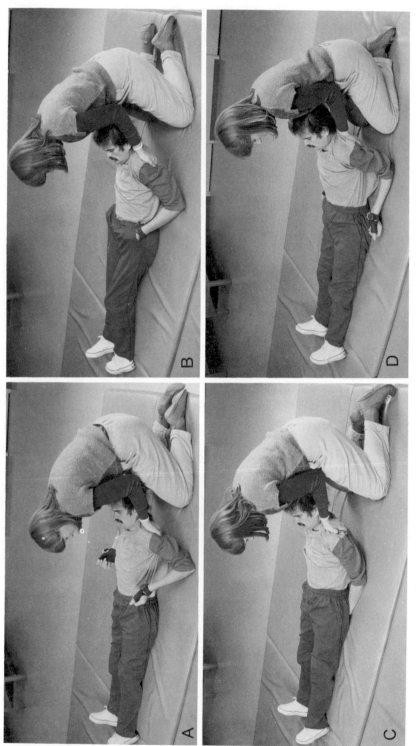

Figure 7.20. A, A person with good shoulder and elbow strength may be able to push directly up into a supine-on-elbow position, using shoulder extensors and scapula retractor muscles. B and C, A person may "fix" his or her hand into the pants pockets or belt loops or under the hips to pull the trunk off the bed. D, The final position is achieved by using the head to initiate the weight shift and "walk" the elbows back until they are under the shoulders.

extended extremity, the patient frees the opposite elbow so it can be positioned in a similar extended posture. The patient can bring the trunk and upper extremities forward to complete long-sitting (Fig. 7.21).

In the long-sitting position, balance activities should be emphasized, with and without using the arms for support (Fig. 7.22). It is important to remember that the low back should not be stretched

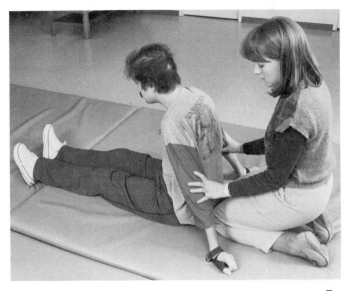

Figure 7.21. The long-sitting position with elbows locked in extension. Tenodesis is maintained in the hand.

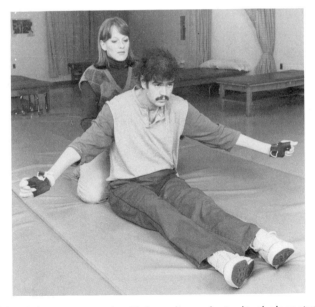

Figure 7.22. Balance activities should always be emphasized in the long-sitting position to prepare the patient for numerous functional activities.

when attempting to balance in this position. Also, the patient with quadriplegia should always maintain tenodesis of the hand when weightbearing through the upper extremities.

The patient should learn to perform push-ups by locking the elbows and depressing the scapula and also learn to manage and position the lower extremities. These activities lead up to transfer, dressing, and self-ROM skills (Fig. 7.23.)

The patient may progress to an *all-fours position* from a long-sitting or prone position (Fig. 7.24). The patient may need assistance to stabilize the hips and feet when assuming this position. In the all-fours position, the patient should concentrate on balance and coordination in preparation for kneeling, front-on approach floor-to-wheelchair transfers, and ambulation activities.

Using the chair, stool, or stall bars for support, a patient may pull him- or herself to kneeling from the all-fours position. Good balance and hip control are important in this position for the patient who is performing floor-to-wheelchair transfers.

Although stability in the long-sitting position is necessary in preparation for certain transfers, bed mobility, self-ROM activities, and dressing, the *short-sitting posture* is equally important for functional activities. Many transfers are performed in the short-sitting position, and good balance is crucial although often difficult to maintain for the patient with quadriplegia.

Short-sitting balance should be stable with and without support of the arms. Even small movements of the head and trunk affect a patient's balance in this position, and the patient should learn the adjustments necessary to maintain balance (Fig. 7.25).

The patient who has at least wrist extensor function should be able to manage the lower extremities when moving from a short-sitting to a supine on bed or mat position (Fig. 7.26). This can be an exhaustive and time-consuming activity for the patient with minimal hand func-

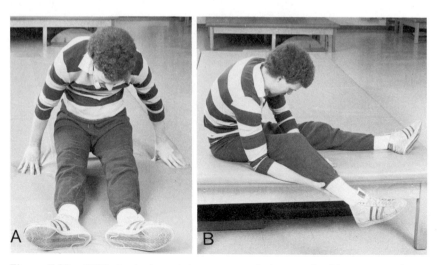

Figure 7.23. While in the long sitting position, the person should attempt push-ups and practice managing the lower extremities in preparation for transfers, dressing activities, and orthoses application.

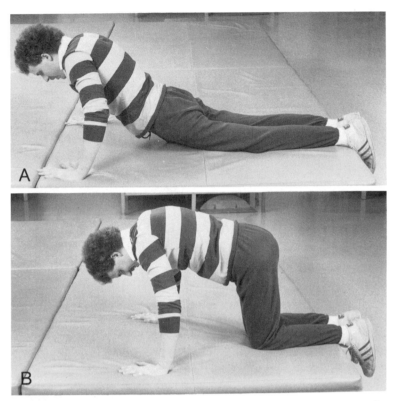

Figure 7.24. Progression to an all-fours (quadriped) position is necessary for the person who will be transferring from the floor to the wheelchair.

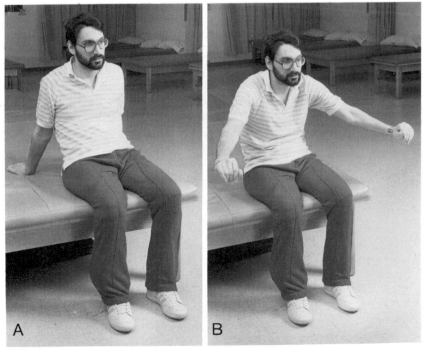

Figure 7.25. Stability in the short-sitting position, with and without support of the arms, is important for transfers and ADL.

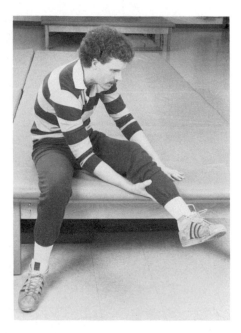

Figure 7.26. Each person will develop his or her own style of getting the legs onto the bed. This activity is easier for the person who has good hand function.

tion. The patient and therapist should try different methods to determine the most efficient technique for the patient. Some patients may find that triggering a spasm is the easiest method of pulling the legs onto the bed or mat.

Activities in the kneeling and sitting positions prepare a patient for *floor-to-wheelchair transfers.* Two different approaches may be used when transferring to or from wheelchair to floor.

The first approach is the front-on method in which a patient begins the transfer from the floor to the chair in the kneeling position. By performing a push-up, the patient can lift the hips and pivot the trunk in a coordinated movement to lift the buttocks onto the seat of the wheelchair (Fig. 7.27). The sequence can be reversed when transferring to the floor from the wheelchair, or the person may choose to transfer head first onto the floor from the chair (Fig. 7.28).

The second method of floor-to-chair transfer requires a great deal of upper body strength and good use of leverage. With the back positioned toward the chair, the patient may reach back for the armrests, legrests and/or wheelchair seat and perform a push-up to lift the buttocks into the chair. To attain a higher lift the patient should tuck the chin and flex the trunk forward. This principle of moving the head and trunk opposite to the desired movement of the hips is very effective for facilitating movement in many of the transfer and mobility activities (Fig. 7.29).

Mat Class. Mat classes should be designed to achieve many of the same goals as an individual treatment program. There are advantages to group classes that should be considered when planning treat-

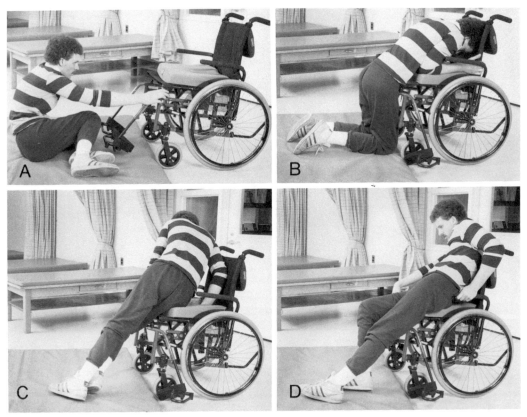

Figure 7.27. The front-on method of floor-to-chair transfer is usually the easier of the methods to learn to get back into the wheelchair. The sequence may be reversed when going to the floor from the wheelchair.

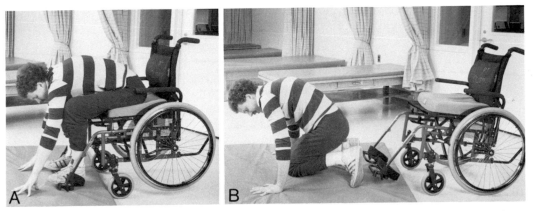

Figure 7.28. A person may prefer to transfer forward to the floor and lower him- or herself slowly with the arms.

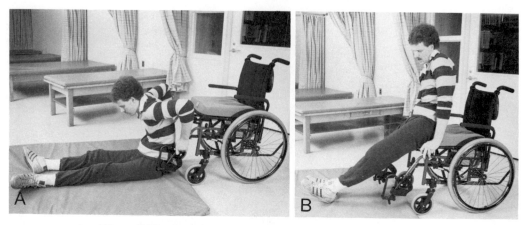

Figure 7.29. Pushing up into the chair from the floor in this manner requires a great deal of upper body strength and relatively long arms. It is often more difficult than the front-on method.

ment programs. Group sessions may motivate patients to compete positively with fellow patients. In addition, patients are able to work on strengthening, coordination, balance, and flexibility during mat group and can then concentrate on special skills and ADL development during the one-on-one sessions. Classes also make economical use of staff time.

Classes may be designed to work on upper or lower extremity strengthening, wheelchair mobility, or ambulation skills.

Self-Range of Motion. When possible, a patient should be taught to range the extremities independently, concentrating on hip, knee, and ankle flexibility. If necessary, a patient may sit against a wall for added support during lower extremity ROM exercises. Having the patient perform self-ROM exercises ensures flexibility maintenance and allows for more efficient use of treatment time to concentrate on specialized skills.

AMBULATION

"When will I be able to walk?" is a question invariably raised by the patient and family members. The decision to brace a patient should be made on an individual basis, and the neurologic level may only play a small part in the decision.

Although it may be a poor principle to brace someone who has an injury higher than a T10 level, many patients go to considerable trouble and expense to find a facility where the staff agrees to brace the patient. Denying the patient an opportunity to prove him- or herself may waste more time than the bracing process itself. It may be more prudent to determine whether bracing is appropriate *by trial, rather than level of injury.*

Patients may need to try temporary lower extremity orthoses to discover for themselves how much energy and time are required. They can then decide if ambulatory or wheelchair locomotion will best suit their needs.

Considerations for Bracing.   The patient should understand the functional limitations of bracing. Braces do not furnish power to the legs, nor is bracing the first step that will eventually lead to "normal" ambulation.

The physiologic effects and benefits of standing and walking related to calcium excretion are still controversial. The issue of energy expenditure during ambulation is also problematic. Studies have demonstrated that a paraplegic patient who ambulates with two knee-ankle-foot orthoses and crutches has an increased oxygen uptake to six times the value for a nonspinal cord injured person and an average velocity less than half the normal ambulation velocity. Quite often after ambulating, the individual is too fatigued to do any other activity.

The patient should know that if assistance is required for donning or doffing the braces or for guarding while ambulating, then he or she will be less independent than without the braces.

Ambulation or "gaiting" demands tremendous physical endurance and a high frustration toleration level. Above-average upper extremity strength is crucial for the patient who now must move the entire trunk and lower extremities with the muscles that normally moved the arms.

To achieve good standing balance, the patient must be free from contractures, especially hip flexion and ankle plantar flexion contractures. Patients who have paralysis of the hip extensor muscles learn to balance on their "Y" (iliofemoral) ligaments and keep their center of gravity posterior to the hip joint to remain upright.

Gaiting is contraindicated before 6 months following fracture stabilization. If the patient should ambulate before this time, a fall may dislodge the stabilization devices.

Orthoses.   There are many options available in orthoses for ambulation. An extensive training period is necessary to determine the most appropriate orthosis for the patient.

The conventional metal *knee-ankle-foot orthosis (KAFO)* uses a double-action ankle joint and offers a choice of knee-locking mechanisms and component parts. The *Craig-Scott KAFO* incorporates stability and balance into the design of the brace by a special shoe structure and a solid ankle joint set in approximately 10° of dorsiflexion. The knee joints are offset ½ inch posterior to the anatomic axis, and a bale locking system provides for automatic locking and unlocking of the knee.

Polypropylene KAFOs can be lighter than the conventional or Craig-Scott KAFOs, but must fit precisely to the patient's legs. Polypropylene orthoses are not indicated for the patient who has fluctuating edema or marked spasticity.

The *LSU reciprocal brace* is molded to the patient's legs and operates on the principle that a patient will use a reciprocal gait pattern. The orthosis uses a dual-cable design by which hip flexion on one side pulls the opposite hip into extension. Comparatively, the LSU orthosis requires a lot of time to apply.

Functional electrical stimulation (FES) may be used as a definitive orthotic device or in conjunction with an orthosis, such as the LSU reciprocal brace. FES can be used during ambulation to stimulate muscles during the swing and stance phases via a heel or hand-triggered switch. Use of FES requires an intensive training period, and not all patients are candidates for FES.

Ideally, ambulation programs using training orthoses allow the patient to experiment with different adjustments and modifications and should precede any definitive orthotic prescription.

Gait Training. On the average, gait training can take from 3–6 weeks or longer, depending on the patient's motor recovery, balance, endurance, and determination. Gait training should begin in the parallel bars and progress to outside the bars once the patient develops balance, weight shifting ability, and control of the trunk and legs during ambulation.

Before ambulating, the patient must develop a "balance point," a three-point base of support that the patient can temporarily maintain without using the arms. The patient should learn how to keep the center of gravity posterior to the hip joint or jack-knifing may occur.

The patient should be taught more than one gait pattern during training in the parallel bars. The *four-point gait pattern* is similar to the normal walking pattern and is the safest gait pattern. In this pattern, the patient always has at least three points of contact on the ground at any time. The four-point gait pattern is useful in tight places, but most patients elect not to use this pattern as it is both time and energy consuming.

Most patients prefer a *swing-to* or *swing-through gait pattern.* The patient swings the feet up to, but not past the point of the crutches, in a swing-to gait and goes beyond the crutch placement in a swing-through pattern. Both gait patterns are easy to learn because they are an extension of the three-point standing posture. These gait patterns

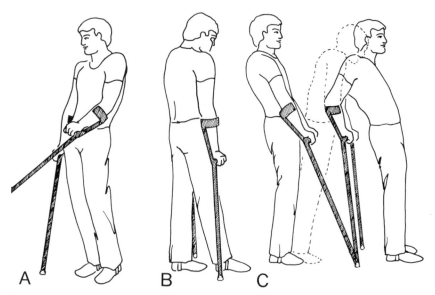

Figure 7.30. *A,* A person must be able to reach a balance point when standing before engaging in ambulation activities. *B* and *C,* Four-point gait patterns, swing-to, or swing-through patterns should be learned.

are faster than the four-point, but the patient must always remember to keep the center of gravity posterior to the hip joint to prevent falling (Fig. 7.30).

Elevation Activities. Ascending and descending stairs with the knees locked in extension may be accomplished by either a forward or backward approach. Training should start on small, wide steps, using one or both railings and then progress to higher levels with railings and/or crutches.

When ascending stairs, the patient should place the crutches on the step above. The crutches should remain on the same step as the patient when descending. The patient must learn to regain the balance position quickly after landing on the next step. A patient gains additional lift if he or she tucks the chin and flexes the trunk forward while pushing down on the crutches (Fig. 7.31).

The technique for managing curbs is similar to those used on the

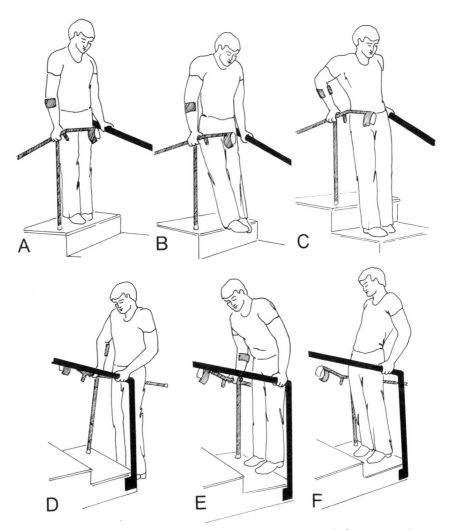

Figure 7.31. A person should learn how to negotiate stairs before progressing to curbs without railings. When stepping up or down, the person must quickly regain the balance point.

stairs. The training should begin on smaller curbs and eventually progress to higher curbs.

Ramps may be approached forward, backward, sideways, or on a diagonal. Steeper inclines require the patient to use a shorter stride and/or swing-to, rather than a swing-through gait pattern. Some patients prefer to negotiate ramps diagonally using a four-point gait pattern.

Transferring to or from the Wheelchair. There are two basic techniques for getting into and out of the wheelchair. In the first method of rising from the chair, the patient locks the knee joints of the orthosis and places the crutches perpendicular to the floor so that his or her elbows are pointing toward the ceiling. In one motion, the patient tucks the head, forcefully pushes down on the crutches, and lifts up to an upright position. As soon as the feet are on the floor, the patient must quickly extend the trunk and get the center of gravity posterior to the hip joints.

The sequence is reversed when sitting in the chair. The patient should back to within 6–8 inches from the front of the chair and then place the hands on the armrest. The patient can tuck the head and jack-knife into the chair. The knees can either remain locked, or the patient can allow the bale locks to catch on the wheelchair seat, which causes the knees to buckle.

The second method of rising from the chair requires less balance and coordination. In this technique, the patient should move forward in the chair and cross one leg over the other. By pushing down on the armrests, the patient pivots to a standing position, facing the wheelchair. The patient can reach for the crutches and position them on his or her arms. Backing away from the chair from this position is often difficult for the patient. The patient may be more successful side-stepping or circling from the chair.

The patient should reverse the sequence when returning to the wheelchair from a front-on approach. (Fig. 7.32).

Falling/Getting Up from the Floor. No matter how stable a patient may appear during ambulation, he or she may fall at one time or another. The patient should be taught how to fall and how to assume the standing position once again from the ground.

If possible, the patient should try to fall forward, breaking the fall with bent arms. The patient should practice releasing the crutches and throwing them clear of his or her body. Initially, falling should be practiced on padded or raised surfaces so it is not so frightening.

The easiest method for getting up off the floor is to transfer back into a chair and then assume the standing position, as previously discussed.

Activities of Daily Living

Previous sections addressed the physical management of the patient in terms of strength, balance, coordination, and mobility. However, there are many other aspects of care in the process of recovery.

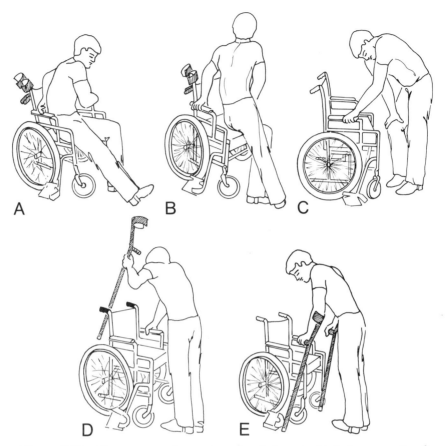

Figure 7.32. This sequence for getting out of the wheelchair in preparation for ambulation may be reversed when sitting down.

Activities of daily living (ADL) encompass the everyday tasks that are necessary for the functional independence of the individual in the home, workplace, and community. These everyday tasks include dressing, hygiene, and feeding, and all aspects of the mobility are incorporated into acquisition of these skills.

DRESSING

Learning to dress in an unconventional manner may be one of the most difficult tasks for the person with quadriplegia. Preparation is a must! The person should have his or her clothes for the following day within reach before going to bed. Doing so eliminates the need to transfer out of bed to get the clothes and back into the bed to dress. Most individuals dress the lower extremities while in bed and the upper extremities while sitting in the wheelchair. Dressing the upper extremities while in the wheelchair provides better support for the patient than dressing in the long-sitting position.

Equipment.   The patient should keep any equipment needed to aid in dressing within reach to avoid any unnecessary maneuvering and energy expenditure.

A dressing stick with a coated coat hook assists the person with pulling and pushing clothing and dressing items and reaching the lower extremities.

Dressing loops made with webbing and an "S" hook may assist with pulling up pants. The person can attach the hook of the dressing loop to loops that may be sewn to the waistband of the pants.

A button hook, adapted to fit on the person's hand, may be necessary for fastening the buttons on a shirt, blouse, or pants for those persons without finger dexterity. A button hook can be further adapted with a hook on the opposite end. The patient can use this hook to pull up the zipper of a jacket or pants. A small key ring or nylon loop of string may be used as a zipper pull, and Velcro may be used to replace buttons or snaps for easy fastening. Figure 7.33 illustrates equipment that may assist the person with quadriplegia with dressing.

UPPER EXTREMITY DRESSING

A person with quadriplegia may find it prudent to change his or her style of clothing when buying new blouses and shirts. Selecting clothing without buttons and thereby eliminating the need for using a button hook saves time in dressing. The clothing material should be durable but easy to wash and wear. Shirts and blouses that can be worn on the outside of pants eliminate the chore of tucking them in.

Donning a Shirt or Blouse. There are several methods for donning a shirt or blouse, and the method chosen will depend on the individual's abilities. A person with good sitting balance and adequate upper extremity strength may be able to don a shirt in the conventional manner by placing one arm into a sleeve and swinging the shirt around to insert the other arm.

An alternative method of donning is to place the shirt on the lap and insert both arms into the sleeves. The sleeves should be pushed above the elbows, and the patient should place the thumbs on the collar. While raising the arms above the head, the patient should duck the head forward to allow the shirt to slip over the head. The person can lean forward making sure to hook one arm over the back of the chair for stabilization and wiggle his or her trunk until the shirt slips down in the back. This method of donning can be used for button-down shirts that have all but the top two or three buttons fastened.

A T-shirt is usually easiest for the person to don. The person can use the over-the-head method and then place the hand inside the shirt to pull it into position once it is over the head. If the patient does not have adequate strength or ROM to pull the shirt over the head, he or she should use a dressing stick to assist with the pull.

Bra Management. Donning a bra seems to present difficulty for the patient as it may roll up. The patient may choose to go braless, rather than deal with the hassles of putting on the bra.

The patient may don a back-hook bra by fastening the bra in front before turning it around, or she may simply choose to wear a front-fastening bra. Loops placed at the fasteners may help the patient hook the bra. Some people prefer to wear a stretch bra instead and not worry about fastening. Stretch bras may be better for the woman with

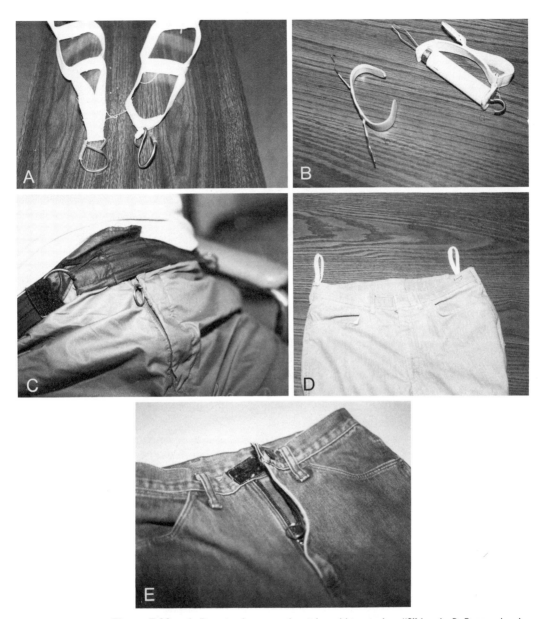

Figure 7.33. *A,* Dressing loops made with webbing and an "S" hook. *B,* Button hooks adapted with a zipper pull on the opposite end. *C,* Key ring placed on zipper to facilitate opening and closing with fingers or hook. *D,* Loops sewn to pants to assist donning. *E,* Velcro used to replace snaps or buttons.

a small breast size. Velcro replacements for fasteners have been known to loosen with vigorous activities and are not recommended.

Removing the Shirt or Blouse. The patient should completely open the button-down shirt before pulling it off the shoulders. The patient should use the stronger arm to pull the shirt off the opposite shoulder and then maneuver the arm out of the sleeve. The shirt then can be pulled around to the other arm and shaken off if necessary. A patient who has good sitting balance may be able to remove a button-down shirt by stabilizing one arm behind the chair and leaning forward to pull the shirt off over the head. A loop sewn into the collar of the shirt makes it easier for the patient to grab onto the collar and pull the shirt over his or her head.

DRESSING LOWER EXTREMITIES

Donning the Pants.   The most common method of donning pants in the early phases of rehabilitation is for the patient to begin in the long-sitting position, either with the head of the bed elevated or with the patient leaning against the headboard. As the individual's balance improves, he or she should be able to dress without back support. The person should toss the pants just beyond his or her feet and position the waist of the pants under each heel. By using the thumbs in the belt loops or using dressing loops, the person should pull the pants toward the buttocks as far as possible. He or she can then fall back to a supine-on-elbow position and alternately shift weight to one side while pulling the pants up as far as possible on the opposite side. It may require several alternate weight shifts to get the pants over the buttocks.

With an improvement in agility and ability, a person may use other positions to don the pants. In a long-sitting position, a patient may alternately bring one knee to the chest and place the foot into the pant leg. Some individuals may be more successful dressing in the wheelchair. A dressing stick may be necessary to assist with donning the pants.

Undressing the Lower Extremities.   For some patients, undressing is more difficult because the clothes tend to gather, especially in creases, and are hard to remove. The person should initially learn to undress while in bed and then may choose to undress in the wheelchair once his or her balance is improved. The patient may remove the pants while in the long-sitting position by placing the thumbs inside the waist and gradually pushing the pants down over the hips, shifting weight from side-to-side until the pants are over the feet. A dressing stick may be used to assist the person with pushing the pants off the leg.

Putting on Socks.   Crew socks are the most suitable type of sock as they stretch, but still maintain their shape. Shoe-string loops may be sewn into the socks so that the individual will be able to place his or her thumbs into the loops and pull the sock.

Support stockings (TEDS) are extremely difficult to apply for the patient without finger function. In the early phases of recovery, the patient may be dependent in donning and removing this type of stocking. Socks should be donned before pants in order to contain the patient's toes while the pants are being pulled over the legs.

Shoes.   Patients should don their shoes while in bed, after donning their socks and pants. While in the long-sitting position, the person may cross one leg over the opposite ankle, which will allow the shoe to slip easily over the foot. A loop sewn on the back of the shoe aids in pulling the shoe over the heel.

For many years, therapists have adapted regular tie shoes with Velcro straps to facilitate donning and removal of the shoe. Shoes that are now commercially available with Velcro fasteners have solved many dressing problems for the patient with quadriplegia. Shoes with elastic strings or slip-on shoes are also easier for the patient to don. Another method to facilitate the donning of shoes is to rivet the shoe tongue at the first shoe string hole (Fig. 7.34). The shoes can be tied loosely, and the patient will be able to slip the foot into the shoe without being hindered by the tongue of the shoe.

HYGIENE

Hygiene training may be initiated as soon as the patient is able to sit in a wheelchair for extended periods of time. The person with paraplegia who has full motor power of the upper extremities should have no difficulty performing hygiene activities. A long-handled bath brush and tub bench (Fig. 7.35) may be the only pieces of adaptive equipment necessary for bathing purposes.

However, the person with quadriplegia must relearn the many aspects of hygiene care so frequently taken for granted by the able-bodied individual.

Washing the Face. The person may balance while washing the face by placing the elbows on the sink counter. He or she may drape a washcloth over the hand and remove excess water from the cloth by pressing it against the inside of the sink. Commercially available soap dispensers usually can be managed by the person with limited grasp function. Long-lever faucet arms are also commercially available, or an orthoplast adaptation can be fabricated to assist the patient with turning the water off and on (Fig. 7.36).

Caring for the Teeth. Caring for the teeth is especially important for the quadriplegic individual who may use the teeth to assist with

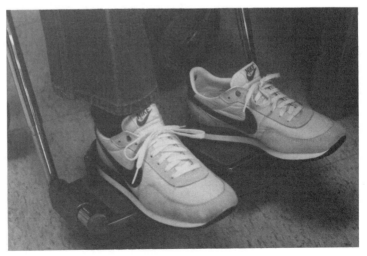

Figure 7.34. Sneakers may be adapted by riveting the shoe tongue at the first shoe string hole to allow the patient to slip the foot into the shoe without hindrance from the shoe's tongue.

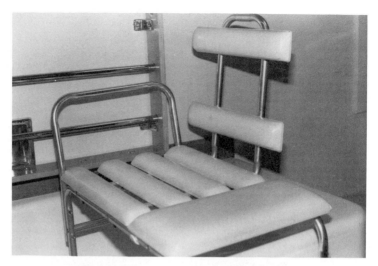

Figure 7.35.   Tub bench used for bathing.

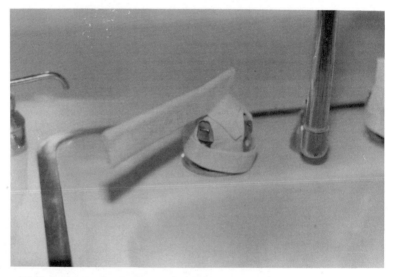

Figure 7.36.   Orthoplast adaptation fabricated to fit the faucet handles assists the person with limited hand functions in hygiene activities.

many self-care activities. The patient may place the toothbrush in a *universal cuff,* of if he or she has a functional tenodesis, a built-up handle may be used for holding the toothbrush. There are several methods of applying the toothpaste. The person could press the tube with the heels of both hands to squeeze the toothpaste onto the brush or directly squeeze the paste into the mouth. Use of the pump tooth-paste dispenser may be the easiest method for applying toothpaste on the brush. The patient should use the teeth and tongue combined with head movements to reposition the brush in the mouth to clean the teeth properly.

The patient who wears dentures may be able to remove them by thrusting the tongue in back of the dentures and pushing them forward. The person should place both hands under the mouth to prevent the dentures from falling onto the floor. Once removed, the person can either place the dentures in a container for cleaning or clean them by using a suction brush attached to the sink.

Shaving. Based on the individual's strength, range of motion, and spasticity, either a straight-edge or electric razor may be used for shaving. The person could place a straight-edge razor in a universal cuff and manipulate the razor in the cuff to shave all areas of this face. He may also use a lightweight electric razor with a Velcro, D-ring attachment if his grasp is limited. If the patient cannot grasp the razor, a gooseneck device may be used with the electric razor mounted on it. Then, by manipulating the wheelchair into various positions, a person may shave his entire face.

Females with quadriplegia experience more difficulty with shaving because of the areas of the body that they shave. Depending on the woman's functional grasp, a straight-edge or electric razor may be used. By placing the elbows on a countertop to maintain balance, the patient could shave one underarm at a time, switching the razor to the hand opposite of the arm to be shaved. The woman should use either an electric razor or commercially available creams to remove hair on the legs.

Deodorant. The patient is most successful using stick deodorants, which can be applied when held in any direction. An orthoplast handle may be attached to the deodorant container for the patient with limited hand function.

Hair Care. Hair care is much easier for the patient who has short or "permed" hair. The patient may be able to wash his or her hair using a hand-held shower head and an adapted palm scrub brush. Shampoos, dispensed from a pump container are more manageable than those from a bottle.

Hand-held dryers that are compact and lightweight and curling irons can be adapted for the patient concerned with a special hair style. The person with limited hand function may not be able to use a curling brush, but may use a brush or comb inserted into a universal cuff or an adapted Velcro D-ring enclosure. Fig. 7.37 illustrates some adapted equipment for hygiene activities.

Makeup Application. Use of makeup may be very important to the female patient, and the therapist and patient can be quite creative in adapting makeup containers for functional use. Tongue depressors can be placed on many containers to facilitate opening and closing them. Extensions can also be mounted on makeup applicators that allow the person to insert them into a universal cuff.

Bathing. Bathing is an important area of hygiene for the individual with a SCI. Depending on functional ability, a patient may bathe in a tub, utilize a tub bench, or wash in a shower that allows the person to use a roll-in shower chair (Fig. 7.38). Use of hand-held showers, long-handled brushes, and bathing mitts allows the person to perform bathing tasks with as little assistance as possible.

Nail Care. Nail care of both hands and feet should be an impor-

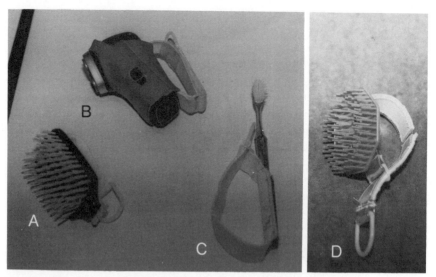

Figure 7.37. D-ring Velcro and universal cuff adaptations for hair brush, razor, and toothbrush. Adapted hair and scrub brush.

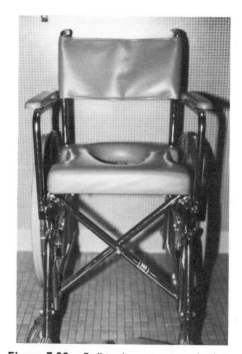

Figure 7.38. Roll-in shower commode chair.

tant consideration for the individual. Ingrown toe nails may cause serious problems, and most patients with quadriplegia are dependent on others for care of the toenails. A nail board can be adapted for hand nail care and used with relative ease. A nail clipper can be firmly mounted to a block of wood, and an extension can be placed on the clipper for the patient to press with the heel of one hand. The patient can simply place the other hand in a position for the nail to be clipped (Fig. 7.39).

Menstrual Management. The woman with either quadriplegia or paraplegia may use sanitary pads during menstruation because the pads do not require good hand function. The patient should place the sanitary pad with the self-adhesive backing in her underpants before donning them. The person who has good finger dexterity and sitting balance should be able to use a tampon and can insert it when seated on a toilet seat, commode chair, or wheelchair. Adaptations for using the tampon are limited, although some individuals may be able to place the tampon into a universal cuff before insertion.

FEEDING

A person who does not have deltoids and biceps muscles will be dependent for feeding. However, it may be possible for the person with tremendous motivation and determination to use a balanced forearm orthosis (BFO) or an overhead sling to suspend the arm, together with a dorsal wrist support splint and utensil pocket, to self-feed. A T-bar that keeps the person's fingers out of the food and a plate guard, which prevents the food from falling off the plate, are also necessary for this task.

Biceps and deltoids function enables the patient to perform the hand-to-mouth movement that is necessary for self-feeding with minimal external assistive devices. The person who does not have wrist extensors needs a dorsal wrist support splint to stabilize the wrist, as well as a utensil pocket or universal cuff for a fork or spoon (Fig. 7.40). If the person has wrist extensor muscles, then only built-up utensil handles or a universal cuff may be needed for placement of the utensils. The fork or spoon may need to be bent for the person to stab the food, and cutting the food is virtually impossible for the person without finger dexterity. A plate guard may also be necessary.

The person who has triceps, wrist flexors, and some finger function should be able to self-feed without assistive devices. A utensil may be held in the normal fashion, or it may be "woven" through the fingers for better stabilization.

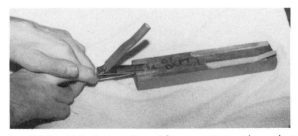

Figure 7.39. Nail clipper adapted for operation with one hand.

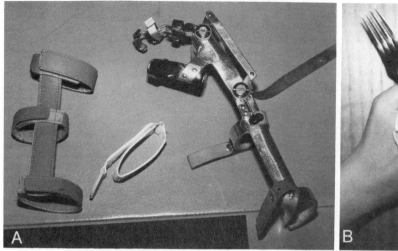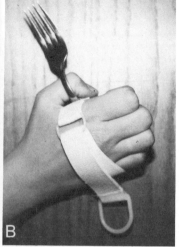

Figure 7.40. *A,* Devices to assist with self-feeding include a dorsal wrist splint, a universal cuff, and a wrist-driven flexor hinge splint. *B,* A fork or spoon can be placed in a universal cuff to assist the person with limited hand function.

Promoting Interaction and Independence

WHEELCHAIR CONSIDERATIONS

A wheelchair can affect a person's mobility, self-care skills, and posture.

Optimally, the fitting process would make available to the patient a fleet of various makes, styles, and options of wheelchairs, allowing the individual to spend time in the chair experimenting with various back heights and seat widths. In most cases, however, a fleet of wheelchairs is not available to the therapist and patient. Therefore, it may be necessary to utilize measurement at designated anatomic locations to determine seat width and back height. The patient's discharge environment should be an important consideration in wheelchair prescription.

Various options deserve special consideration:

1. *Back height:* The back height should give adequate support, yet be low enough to permit sufficient shoulder mobility.

2. *Seat width:* The seat width should be as narrow as possible, thereby keeping the overall width of the wheelchair narrow. There should be at least one finger's width of space between the greater trochanter and the skirt/clothing guard.

3. *Tires:* Pneumatic tires with tread give a better ride and also provide some friction for those who use the wheel to propel.

4. *Casters:* Eight-inch casters are appropriate for all activities except basketball and tennis. There are a variety of caster wheels, including pneumatic, polyurethane, urethane, and hard rubber. The polyurethane and urethane types are the most popular because they give the smooth ride of the pneumatic wheels, but eliminate the problems of flat tires.

5. *Legrests:* Either swing-away or non-swing-away legrests are avail-

able. The individual's abilities and the discharge environment help determine the appropriate legrest.

6. *Armrests:* Armrests can be removable or nonremovable. Removable armrests should be the choice of the majority of patients, allowing the removal of the armrest for transfers if necessary. Even the individual who does not remove the armrest for transfers may at some time need this option.

Table 7.1
Commercially Available Cushions

Cushions	Comments
Roho Dry Floatation Cushion	Neoprene rubber base with a system of interconnected flexible air cells Even weight distribution Low surface tension Can tie down individual cells to decrease pressure on specific areas
Jobst	Particles of foam in liquid that forms a gel Heavy Slick nylon cover that allows some patients to slip forward in chair
Jay	Flolite pad with molded urethane foam base Scooped-out area in rear Sometimes difficult to transfer out of wheelchair Provides even pressure May be used in car Decreased shearing force Enhances posture
T-Foam	Visco-elastic foam Three densities and thickness Contours to body shape Low shearing Lightweight
Foam	Polyurethane foam Several sizes Lightweight Fire retardant Machine washable Nomex cloth cover
Combi	Posture seating system Molded from two types of foam—firm support foam and outside layers of softer foam for comfort Waterproof cover available Nonskid bottom Scooped-out area, possibly making transfers difficult Contoured backrest (lumbar pad)
Laminaire	Two types of premium-grade polyurethane foam Available with sacral cut-out Lightweight polyester knit cover

CUSHIONS

There are numerous cushions on the market, and care should be taken to select the cushion most suitable for the individual. Cushion materials include foam, gel, water, rubber or their combination.

Some of the more popular cushions are described in Table 7.1.

ENVIRONMENTAL CONTROL UNITS

Environmental control units (ECU) allow the person with paralysis of the upper extremities to gain some control of the immediate environment. Electronically designed systems permit the patient to perform such tasks as turning on the lights, answering the telephone, and turning on the radio or television set. The person who can only move his or her head may operate an ECU by using a sip-and-puff device. If the person has limited upper extremity function, a rocker control mechanism may be used to activate the unit (Fig. 7.41).

COMMUNICATION SKILLS

Writing and/or typing skills and the ability to use a telephone are necessary functions for most vocational and avocational pursuits. The person with quadriplegia should be given every opportunity to be able to develop these skills.

Writing Activities. There are many adaptations that a person can use who does not have finger movement. A patient who has a functional tenodesis may be able to write using a built-up pen with rubber tubing or by lacing the pen through the fingers. Felt tip pens that do not require as much pressure as ballpoint pens are recommended for patient use.

Adaptive writing splints are required for the person with limited hand function. There are different styles available that place the hand in a typical position for writing. The person needs practice to develop writing speed and legibility using the devices. Some of the available devices are a universal cuff with a right-angle attachment for the pen

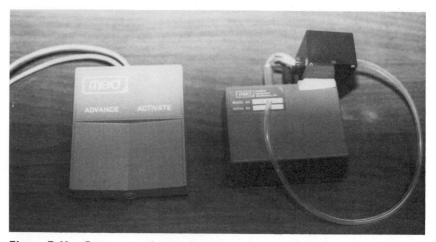

Figure 7.41.   Environmental control units may be controlled using a "rocker" mechanism (*left*) or by a "sip-and-puff" device.

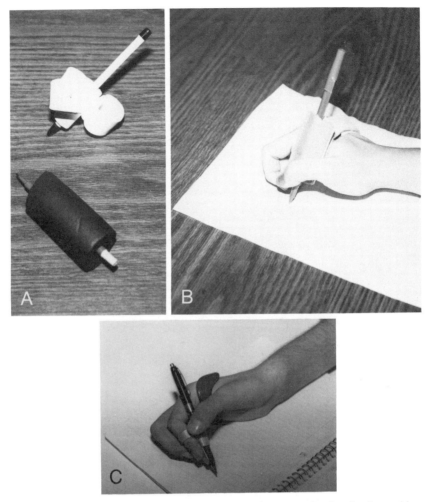

Figure 7.42. *A,* Adaptations for writing can be made using orthoplast (*top*) or rubber tubing to build up pens for the person with a functional tenodesis. *B,* Right-angle attachment to universal cuff for pen insert. *C,* Wanchik writing splint.

insert, a Wanchik writing splint; a wrist-driven flexor hinge splint for the patient who has wrist extensors, and, an orthoplast splint (Fig. 7.42).

Typing. Typing is the most effective means of written communication for the person with quadriplegia above a C5 level. Suspension slings, ball-bearing feeders, and mouthsticks can be used to assist the person with this activity. The mouthpiece of a mouthstick should be fabricated by a dentist to ensure proper fit. In addition, the person should always have a mouthstick holder within reach to allow for periods of rest (Fig. 7.43). The person may operate the typewriter using the mouthstick, with the eraser end of a pencil, or with a dowel stick with a rubber tip inserted into a universal cuff if hand function permits (Fig. 7.44).

Telephone Skills. The telephone should be stabilized to prevent movement when dialing. The patient should be able to dial the push-

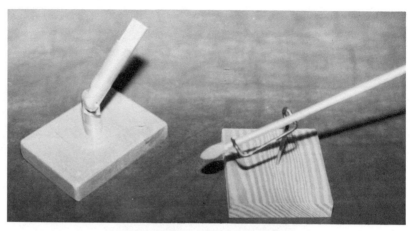

Figure 7.43. Mouthstick holders.

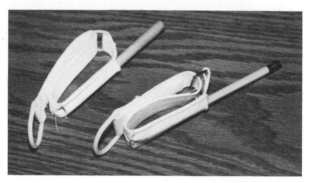

Figure 7.44. A dowel stick (*left*) or the eraser end of a pencil may be inserted into a universal cuff to assist the person who has minimal hand function with typing activities.

button phone by using the same device used for typing. Telephones that have a memory bank require only one button to push to dial a number and are best suited for the patient with quadriplegia. The higher-level quadriplegic patient may need a speaker phone or may use an ECU to operate the telephone.

Managing the receiver may present a problem for the person with poor hand function. An orthoplast adaptation may be placed on the receiver that allows the patient to be independent in using the phone. A gooseneck adaptation can be set up to hold the receiver for the person using the phone. A special lever attached to the gooseneck depresses the receiver button when the phone is not in use (Fig 7.45).

DRIVING

Driving offers the individual with SCI a means of freedom, allowing the person to pursue leisure-time interests, as well as providing a means for returning to a work/school environment.

The individual with an injury to C4 or higher is usually unable to drive. It is important, however, that a vehicle be properly equipped to transport the person. Vans or minivans can be equipped with an

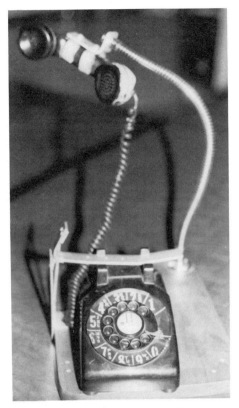

Figure 7.45. A gooseneck adapter used to hold the receiver for the person using the phone. A special lever is adapted to depress the receiver button when the phone is not in use.

electric or hydraulic lift and a tie-down system for securing the wheelchair. The person should also be secured in the wheelchair with a chest strap. The floor of the van should be leveled with plywood or carpet to permit easy maneuvering, and the roof may need to be raised if the individual is taller than 53 inches from the floor when seated in the wheelchair. Because of the patient's sensory loss, rear heaters are also recommended.

The person with a C5 level of injury may be able to drive independently using sensitized equipment—reduced effort/zero braking and steering—or power steering and brakes. The person drives the vehicle while sitting in the wheelchair. For this reason, a drop-pan in the driver's area with an electric tie-down system is necessary for proper positioning and securing of the wheelchair. The driver should wear a chest strap to prevent loss of balance when turning. A console needs to be installed with adapted levers to control the various components normally mounted on the dash board (Fig. 7.46). The console may be mounted either on the driver's door or between the driver's and passenger's seats. Power windows are also recommended. The person who is driving independently also needs a control box mounted outside the van in order to open the door and operate the lift (Fig. 7.47).

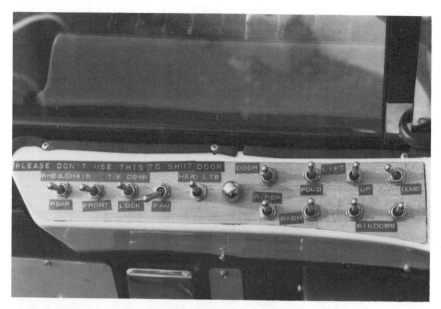

Figure 7.46. A console may be adapted with levers to control the various components normally mounted on the dashboard.

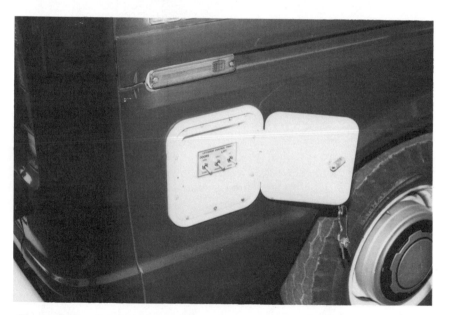

Figure 7.47. A control box needs to be mounted outside the van to control the door and operate the lift.

Various steering devices are available for the patient with different levels of hand function. They include the tri-post, quad grip, and steering knob (Fig. 7.48). The person should select the steering device that is most comfortable and safe for his or her level of injury.

A person whose level of injury is C6 or below should have sufficient strength to drive a vehicle with power steering and brakes. Individuals at this level of injury usually prefer a van to a car because loading the chair into a car is often difficult.

The person who drives a van may or may not be able to transfer into the driver's seat for operating a vehicle. If transfer into the driver's seat is desirable, a six-way power seat is recommended for better positioning and ease of transferring from the wheelchair into the seat.

An individual with an injury below the C6 level should be able to use standard hand controls with power steering and brakes in a car or van. The person should be able to transfer and load the chair independently. Steering devices, such as a steering knob, may be required if the person has difficulty turning the wheel with the palm. [An electric chair top carrier (Fig. 7.49) can be utilized to load the wheelchair on top of the car.]

A citizen band radio is a useful piece of equipment for the car or

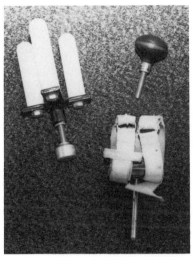

Figure 7.48. Various steering devices, such as the (*clockwise, beginning on left*) tri-post, steering knob, and quad grip, are available to fit the different levels of hand function.

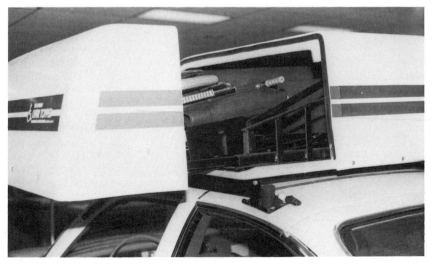

Figure 7.49. An electric car top carrier may facilitate loading/unloading of the wheelchair for the person who prefers to drive a car.

Table 7.2
Functional Levels in Spinal Cord Injury

Level of Injury	Motion Available	Possible Functions
C3	None to little diaphragm Neck motion	Totally dependent in self-care Operate special adapted electric wheelchair with head, mouth, neck, or breath control to propel chair; wheelchair needs portable ventilation system Use mouth stick with maximal assisted setup to type, use tape recorder, calculator, telephone, turn pages, and write Use various types of switches to control stereo, radio, i.e., "sip-and-puff" switch on an environmental control
C4	Neck motion Shoulder elevation	Totally dependent in self-care Operate special adapted electric wheelchair with head, mouth, neck, or breath control to propel chair and independent pressure relief Use mouthstick to perform same functions as listed above Use various types of switches to control environment
Weak C5	Shoulder motions with scapular instability Elbow flexion	Feed self and do light hygiene using adapted equipment Requires maximum to moderate assistance to transfer using a sliding board Maximal assistance with lower extremity dressing using equipment Operate typewriter, telephone, calculator, and tape recorder Push chair short distances on level surfaces; may require electric chair for extended distances and outdoor terrain Possibly can drive using sensitized equipment (zero effort) Able to do independent pressure reliefs
Strong C5	Same motions available as the weak C5 but stronger	Same abilities as a weak C5 but activities are easier Better balance and ability to push and maneuver the

Table 7.2—*continued*

Level of Injury	Motion Available	Possible Functions
		wheelchair; may need electric chair for outdoors or vocational pursuit Requires minimal assistance for transfers Requires moderate to minimal assistance in lower extremity dressing, bathing, bowel and bladder care Can drive using sensitized equipment or possibly power steering/braking Able to do independent pressure reliefs in wheelchairs
C6	Shoulder and scapula motion Elbow flexion Wrist extension providing a tenodesis motion ability for limited prehension without active finger motion	Eating, grooming, hygiene, transfers, upper and lower extremity dressing, pressure relief, writing, typing, etc., and driving (may require a van with lift if unable to load wheelchair in car) Probably able to do independent bathing and bowel and bladder care with adapted equipment Can do cooking and light housework Can wheel chair for longer distances over more difficult terrain; possibly up small curbs With work and motivation can live independently
C7	Shoulder and scapular motion Elbow flexion Elbow extension provided by triceps Wrist extension providing a tenodesis motion ability for limited prehension without active finger motion Wrist flexion Limited finger flexion and extension	Able to do all of the activities that are listed for a C6 but with greater ease Wheeling on outdoor terrain is easier Able to go up and down small curbs Driving may not require a van because it will be somewhat earier for the patient to get a chair into the car Can do cooking and light housework Can live independently
C8	Has all motions in upper extremities except the intrinsic muscles of the hands, causing a weak, imbalanced grasp and decreased fine finger coordination	Able to do the same activities as a C7 Can live independently doing all activities except heavy housework

Table 7.2—*continued*

Level of Injury	Motion Available	Possible Functions
T1	Upper extremities should be innervated; may have a weaker grasp	Can function independently from a wheelchair as a paraplegic Ease of activities is limited due to decreased balance compared with lower level injuries
T2–T5	Increased respiratory functioning with increased costal innervation	Independent from a wheelchair Possible household ambulator with long leg braces
T6–T12	Increased abdominal muscle functioning All abdominal muscles intact in lesions below T12	Independent from a wheelchair T12 has potential for being a functional gaiter with long leg braces if there is strong motivation; may use a combination of gaiting and the wheelchair
L2	Has hip hikers and flexors	Independent from a wheelchair With good motivation much easier for a person at this level to become independent gaiter
L2–L5	Increasing motion in quadriceps and knee motions	In order to ambulate requires various types of bracing to support knee, ankle, and foot or ankle and foot, depending on motor power available
S1–S2	Lower extremity motor power intact except for some motor power in foot	Needs minimal bracing for gaiting

a From Christenson LR: Level of functioning and possible adaptive equipment presented to team members of the Virginia SCI System, Woodrow Wilson Rehabilitation Center.

van in the case of breakdowns and is recommended for all people who will be driving independently.

Table 7.2 summarizes the anticipated functional levels in spinal cord injury and may be used as a reference for the clinician.

HOME MODIFICATIONS

Proper home modification should be an integral part of the rehabilitation process if the individual is to function at his or her maximum potential after discharge.

At a very early stage in the rehabilitation program, a home assessment should be done to determine necessary architectural modifications. This assessment is also important for planning the rehabilitation program. The home environment can be simulated in therapy, thereby allowing the individual to practice the types of activities that may be encountered after discharge.

Through combined expertise of the occupational therapist, physical therapist, and rehabilitation engineer, appropriate equipment recommendations and modifications and suggestions for implementing architectural changes can be offered. Involving a representative of the insurance carrier in the home assessment may facilitate payment for needed modifications.

COMMUNITY RE-ENTRY

Physical needs, such as transfers, dressing, and driving, are very important aspects of the patient's functional existence. Equally important, however, are the individual's needs and concerns about returning to the community. The program of *community re-entry*, mainstreaming the individual into the community, should be geared to the individual's level of independence and community interests.

For the C4 quadriplegic patient, an appropriate re-entry task may be to hire an attendant. Other re-entry tasks may address a person's ability to function in the church community or work/school environment.

Before discharge, the patient should be given information about community resources available to the disabled individual. Addressing an individual's concerns with regard to community re-entry is vital for a smoother adjustment to the community.

Summary

With appropriate training and rehabilitation, the individual with a SCI should be able to return to a functional life-style as a contributing member of the community. The recognition and understanding of the individual's needs when planning the rehabilitation program will ultimately result in an optimal level of independence. The rehabilitation goals can only be achieved through the combined efforts of the patient, family, and rehabilitation team.

Suggested Readings

Bajd T, Kralj A, Turk R, Benko H, Sega J: The use of the four channel electrical stimulator as an ambulatory aid for the paraplegic patient. *Phys Ther* 63:1116–1120, 1983.

Basmajian JE, Kirby RL: *Medical Rehabilitation.* Baltimore, Williams & Wilkins, 1984.

Cerny K, Waters R, Hislop H, Perry J: Walking and wheelchair energetics. *Phys Ther* 60:1133–1139, 1980.

Cull JF, Hardy RE: *Physical Medicine and Rehabilitation Approaches in Spinal Cord Injury.* Springfield, IL, Charles C. Thomas, 1977.

Ford J, Duckworth B: *Physical Management for the Quadriplegic Patient.* Philadelphia, FA Davis, 1974.

Hoberman M, Cicenia EF, Dervitz HL, Sampson O: The use of lead-up exercises to supplement mat work: Exercises without apparatus or equipment. *Phys Ther Rev* 31:321–328, 1951.

Huitt CT, Gwyer JL: Paraplegia ambulatory training using Craig-Scott orthoses. *Phys Ther* 58:976–978, 1978.

Nixon V: *Spinal Cord Injury*. Rockville, MD, Aspen Systems Corp, 1985.

Penjabi M, White AA: Spinal braces: Functional analysis and clinical application. In *Clinical Biomechanics of the Spine*, Philadelphia, JB Lippincott, 1978.

Pierce DS, Nickel VH: *The Total Care of Spinal Cord Injuries*. Boston, Little, Brown and Company, 1977.

Rusk HA: *Rehabilitation Medicine*, ed. 4. St. Louis, CV Mosby, 1977.

Trieschmann RB: *Spinal Cord Injuries: Psychological, Social and Vocational Adjustment*. New York, Pergamon Press, 1982.

Trombly CA: *Occupational Therapy for Physical Dysfunction*, ed 2. Baltimore, Williams & Wilkins, 1983.

CHAPTER 8

Psychosocial Issues and Approaches

BYRON WOODBURY, Ph.D.
CATHY REDD, Ph.D.

This chapter describes the psychological processes commonly experienced by newly injured spinal cord patients from the onset of trauma through re-entry into the community. Psychological concerns and problems generally encountered by this patient population and psychological treatment interventions used to assist patients' coping are addressed in this discussion. At this time, no single theory of response to crisis or adjustment to disability seems to account adequately for the total picture of the patient's psychological process. However, there are a number of theories that provide useful perspectives to consider. These are described briefly.

The purpose of this chapter is to provide allied health professionals with information about the psychological processes associated with onset of spinal cord injuries and to describe the goals and techniques of intervention by psychologists treating these patients. It is not a comprehensive review of all the psychological variables and psychological principles involved in treatment and is not intended to train allied health professionals to provide psychological services to spinal cord injured patients.

During the past 40 years, hundreds of research studies have been published on the psychological aspects of spinal cord injury (SCI). The reader is referred to works by Woodbury (1), Treischmann (2), and Crewe and Krause (3) for comprehensive reviews of research on SCI.

Psychological processes, treatment goals, and interventions are discussed in a sequence that roughly follows the chronology of treatment from acute care through discharge from rehabilitation and to reintegration into the community. Although it is possible in this way to introduce a general order and sequencing of events and concerns, it must be emphasized that each patient must be understood and treated individually.

Each person who is spinal cord injured becomes fully aware of the various issues related to the injury and its effect on future living at a different point in the treatment process. Each person has unique approaches to coping and problem solving. Each person presents his or her own pattern of difficulties and distress over the years following the onset of injury.

Important information about the psychological treatment needs of this population may be obtained by examining the demographic characteristics of the group. Eighty percent of these patients are male. The mean age is 23. The most frequent causes of injury are vehicular accidents, falls, diving accidents, gunshot wounds, person-to-person contact, and medical complications. Most patients describe themselves as physically active, often athletic, and accustomed to physical labor.

It can be seen from the patient population demographics that SCI patients are generally in the adolescent or early adult stages of development. The field of developmental psychology specifies several critically important tasks to be accomplished during these periods of maturation. First, each individual must come to terms with the process of physical maturation and expression, self-concept, and esteem through physical activities. Personal identity is clarified as philosophical, religious, political, and moral stands are taken. Emotional independence and separation from parents are part of an important struggle that must be completed. At the same time, the individual is required to master the norms of socially appropriate behavior. It is generally a stressful time of development. Dreams of the world as it should be, which are acquired in childhood, collide with experiences in the real world. Perceptions and beliefs are altered. In addition, major life decisions are being made. A vocational choice must be planned, and any preparation through education or training must be identified. Choices regarding sexuality and marriage are usually made during this period. By the time early adulthood is reached, many individuals are faced with the stress of parenthood and the development of life in the world of work. Given the general youth of this group, many are likely to be inexperienced in handling a life crisis outside the protective relationships of their family. Many persons become spinal cord injured at a time when they have a limited repertoire of behavioral and emotional tactics for coping with extended crisis.

All of these characteristics and factors have an impact on the psychological needs and treatment of these patients. Every significant developmental task that has been faced or accomplished before injury must be readdressed and re-evaluated in the process of adjustment to life with a SCI.

Acute Phase

Traditionally, rehabilitation for SCI patients started only when the acute medical phase of care was completed. However, the current trend in comprehensive SCI rehabilitation is clearly toward beginning rehabilitation efforts as soon as possible after injury. This has meant the introduction of physical, occupational, and speech, as well as psychology and social work therapy, into intensive care units. Rehabilitation philosophies and attitudes are being shared with patients from the very start of their lives as spinal cord injured individuals. Such early interventions help in the prevention of unnecessary complications, such as bedsores and contractures, and facilitate early gains in mobility and activities of daily living (ADL). This aggressive approach has also caused some reassessment of assumptions about psychological adjustment to SCI during the period immediately following injury.

In the past, most of the psychological literature has minimized the importance of the early stages of injury. The patient was assumed to be in a state of shock or denial (4, 5), with little meaningful emotional change or adaption being accomplished. No doubt, for some unconscious or seriously multiply injured patients this assumption is valid. However, more recent clinical experience (6) seems to support the notion that the process of psychological adjustment begins quite early and early interventions make a significant difference in both the short- and long-term adjustment process.

Often, persons with SCI do not remember much of their acute

care treatment. Although specific memories are lost, however, some basic emotional learning seems to survive this early period. Specifically, patients seem to learn whether the treatment system can be trusted, they are able to retain generally positive expectancies, and the early presentation of factual information seems to engender a greater sense of control in the individual. Although psychological treatment in the acute phase has not been scientifically researched, clinical impressions suggest that early intervention helps a patient progress more rapidly through later rehabilitation with less psychological disruption.

EARLY ADJUSTMENT FACTORS

The primary psychological feature of the initial phase of treatment for traumatic SCI is adjustment to very sudden and massive change. One moment the individual is involved with a job, family, recreation, and all the myriad details of life; the next, he or she is involved in fighting for survival, experiencing pain, tolerating hospital procedures, and attempting to comprehend paralysis. Very few human beings are prepared for such rapid change on such a massive scale. Perhaps the easiest way to see this change is in the labels commonly used in our culture; in one moment an individual goes from being a "person" to being a "patient."

As a patient with SCI, an adult experiences an incredible loss of control. Depending on the level of injury, the person may need help to breathe, eat, talk, eliminate, bathe, dress, move, summon help, cough, and all the other activities we so succinctly cluster together as the "activities of daily living" (ADL). As a person, one has control over the environment, makes choices, experiences the consequences of these choices and, in general, muddles through. However, as an SCI patient, one is totally at the mercy of strangers. This dependency, which is maximized during acute care, ranges from activities absolutely essential to life to all of the small details of comfort and convenience that help to make life bearable. Even in the best of situations, such a loss of control would be extremely difficult for an adult to cope with, but acute care is far from the best of situations.

For most people, an intensive care unit (ICU) is a totally unknown environment. One is placed in a whole room full of exotic instruments attached to one's body in unusual and often painful ways, which make noise, sound alarms, and generally change constantly. Obviously, these instruments are important—that is, everyone checks them—but what they mean is not at all obvious. When medical personnel attempt to explain their function, it is like hearing a foreign language made up of English, Latin, and abbreviations. Of course, there is very little time for explanations. The pace of an ICU tends to be rather frantic and is constant around the clock; the cast of characters is quite large and includes nurses, many different doctors, respiratory therapists, laboratory technicians, and a host of others.

In addition, this totally new environment also includes a strange bed—it may rock, spin, flip, fold, or do other actions—an almost endless variety of tests, procedures, and treatments; and a variety of people asking one to do actions that turn out to be impossible.

Very few people would have the resources to deal effectively with this loss of control and the new environment when they were at their best, but of course, no new SCI patient is at his or her best. First, there may be a good deal of pain involved both in the original injury and its subsequent treatment. Pain clearly interferes with judgment and tolerance. Second, to deal with the pain and other aspects of SCI, patients often receive a great deal of medications that may affect the CNS in general and cognition in particular. Third, often the individual must cope with a great deal of fear, which can have the power to overwhelm even the strongest person. Fourth, the individual is often very tired. Many patients describe very poor sleep with frequent interruptions for turns, medications, vital sign checks, etc. When they are able to sleep, they may experience vivid and frightening nightmares that leave them even more exhausted than before they slept.

Finally, an SCI patient in the acute stage is often cut off from the normal means of coping with stress or change. Getting away from the situation is impossible, quiet contemplation is difficult at best, and the usual sources of counsel are usually unavailable. Pain, medication, fear, fatigue, and isolation all combine for the newly injured SCI patient to virtually ensure that he or she will have psychological difficulty with the loss of control, new environment and, perhaps most crucial, his or her prognosis.

PSYCHOLOGICAL REACTIONS IN THE ACUTE PHASE

Much has been written about the acute psychological adjustment to SCI, but very little research has actually been conducted. The phenomenon of regression is perhaps one of the clearest early consequences of SCI. Various authors have described regression as becoming more child-like and dependent (3), losing control (7), losing reinforcement (8), becoming egocentric (9), and becoming focused on more basic levels of need. To some extent, all of these descriptions can be applied with a fair degree of accuracy to newly injured individuals.

In the very early time after injury (48–72 hr) the process of regression can be directly observed in the alert and oriented patient. The questions that individuals ask tend to reflect their concerns. Initially, they may refer to their jobs, upcoming appointments, and future events; when they can return home; and so on.

As the seriousness of the situation becomes more clear, the issues of importance become more basic and immediate. Questions about dying, eating, sleeping, obtaining a nurse, and prognosis become more frequent. From a psychological viewpoint, this is regression. Unfortunately, our culture tends to apply a negative connotation to regression. Yet, as shall be seen, regression serves a useful and important function in enabling the individual to adjust psychologically to spinal cord injury. It provides an individual with the ability to tolerate, to some extent, the overwhelming loss of control, the unknown environment, and personal distress described above. It enables a person to pull back and regroup so that he or she can then move toward adjustment as adaptively as possible.

Yet, all SCI patients do not react in a similar manner. Despite similar issues to be faced and similar tasks to be mastered, every person with a SCI has a unique fund of experience upon which to draw. The newly injured individual may not follow any of the carefully thought out models of adjustment. Instead, the patient is likely to approach this brand new situation in the manner that seems to be the best to him or her and will make the best efforts possible toward adjustment. Injured persons may keep to themselves, or they may be painfully public in their efforts. Certainly, some efforts are more adpative than others, but health care professionals always need to remain aware that there is no one "right" way to go about adjusting to SCI. Our job is to facilitate the patient's progress, not dictate it. Strangely enough, this issue becomes more relevant for more experienced professionals. After working with many SCI patients, it becomes difficult to remember that no matter how many times the professional has been through the adjustment process with other patients, this is the first time for this patient.

In addition to regression, various other common early reactions to traumatic SCI have been observed. One of the most useful approaches to this phase is Meyerson's (10) work on unknown situations. Extending earlier work by Lewin (11), Meyerson predicts common patient behavior based upon known reactions to unknown situations. When people are placed in an unknown situation, they are faced with the need to interact with an environment they do not understand in a manner they have never learned. In learning theory terms, they have not learned the behavioral sequence that will lead to predictable reinforcement—that is, goal attainment—from the environment. There are several predictable consequences of being in an unknown situation.

First, the individual does not know where the environmental rewards are located. As a result, efforts to secure rewards will be haphazard, tentative, and idiosyncratic. If one doesn't know where one is going, it is impossible to go there directly. A more concrete example is that the patient who does not understand the negative consequences of contractures is not likely to pursue the sometimes painful but necessary steps to avoid them. Because the person's efforts are not direct or clear-cut, that person is quite likely to become frustrated, angry, and "manipulative." Without an outlet for these feelings, the person is likely to internalize the anger and become depressed. However, if the person has a clear sense of progress toward a clear goal, there may be no negative reaction at all.

If the person's first efforts at structuring the unknown situation are unsuccessful, his or her behavior is likely to become more extreme. If pushing the call light does not bring a nurse, then perhaps yelling will, and if yelling doesn't, perhaps throwing things will, and if throwing doesn't. ... Because structuring the unknown is so important psychologically, the only limits to extreme behavior are the patient's imagination and the staff's tolerance. An understanding of what the patient is trying to accomplish can usually help reduce and eliminate extreme behavior.

Another predictable response to an unknown situation is *hypersensitivity* to small cues. When one does not understand the environment, everything is potentially important. Every alarm could mean disaster, a therapist's expression and comments could be crucial, a nurse's mood could mean danger, anything could mean anything. Without some way to discriminate the important from the trivial, the patient tries to absorb it all (and there is definitely too much to absorb). The most commonly observed consequence of hypersensitivity is the patient's clinging to an established routine and resisting even positive changes of unknown meaning. It is far safer to stick with the known than to accept change and all of the new unknown cues that change may bring.

Unknown situations tend to put people into *approach-avoidance conflicts*. On the one hand, a person wishes to master the unknown and learn the required behavior. On the other hand, unknown situations are inherently uncomfortable, and the desire to escape them is strong. As a result, a newly injured person is likely to fluctuate between working hard and not working at all. This behavioral change may be rapid and extreme. The individual will shift back and forth in both directions, but gradually will do so less often. As with all persons in conflict, the person with SCI will also experience emotional lability and self-doubt.

For some patients, the combination of the psychological and medical aspects of SCI is simply too much to bear. In one study (2), 16% of newly injured SCI patients experienced a brief psychotic episode within the first 2 weeks of injury. Fortunately, the majority of these episodes lasted less than a full day and did not appear to cause long-term problems. It is probably a testament to human resiliency that these episodes are so brief and relatively infrequent.

Two other psychological reactions of newly injured SCI patients have received considerable attention in the literature. They are *depression* and *denial*, and both warrant special attention due to the controversy and common misperceptions surrounding them.

Depression.   Depression is very often written about in the psychological literature, but is seldom rigorously researched. It is often cited as a normal consequence of SCI (12, 13) and plays a major role in many stage theories of adjustment (14, 15). According to these theories some period of depression is necessary for a healthy adjustment to SCI, and conversely, an individual who does not display depression is avoiding dealing with important aspects of reality and thus will not become "adjusted." This view is entirely consistent with knowledge gained from experience with psychiatric populations and a psychodynamic theoretical orientation. Unfortunately, the population who becomes spinal cord injured is not a psychiatric population for the most part and displays very little classic psychopathology.

Research on SCI population samples has strongly challenged traditional concepts about the role of depression. Several personal descriptions of adjustment minimize the role of depression (8, 16, 17), several research efforts have failed to demonstrate a major role for depression in adjustment (18, 19), and at least two studies have found depression to be negatively related to positive adjustment (20, 21).

That is, people who exhibit a lot of depression do not do very well after they are discharged from rehabilitation.

It is difficult to know what to make of these very different findings. Clinically, SCI patients often (but not always) show signs of depression. They are withdrawn and tearful, they say they are depressed, and they have difficulty sleeping and eating. However, they usually continue to work in therapy and make reasonable progress.

Part of the problem in interpreting these findings seems to be in our understanding of depression. It is increasingly clear that depression is not a unitary phenomenon. Various authors have characterized depression as internalized anger, sadness over loss, loss of reinforcers, learned helplessness, and result of biochemical change (4, 15, 22, 23). It is probable that the signs of depression seen in various SCI patients represent a range of meanings, and once again, each patient is unique. For one person depression may be a period of marshalling strength to go on, for another it may be sinking into failure, and for still another depression may never occur. Each case requires a careful understanding of the individual involved and the meaning of the observed behaviors.

Another possible aspect that clouds our understanding of depression is the change in treatment approaches over time. Most of the literature emphasizing the role of depression is older than the literature that de-emphasizes its role. Dr. George Hohmann, a psychologist who became spinal cord injured at the close of World War II, describes the experience of receiving his prognosis:

> When I was injured 32 years ago, I was jolly well depressed, as I look back on it, because I was told that I would never have a family—I was told that I would be in an institution for the remainder of my life, and the expectations were set by the institution and by their prevailing knowledge (2).

Fortunately. Dr. Hohmann and others went out into the world and demonstrated that individuals with SCI can work, play, marry, raise families, and lead independent lives of high quality. As a result, newly injured SCI patients are now given much different messages during acute care. They are told of others' successes and are usually given some positive expectancies from the earliest period of their injury. It is at least possible that this change in approach over time has truly changed the nature of depression following a traumatic SCI.

Denial. Like depression, the concept of *denial* has received considerable attention in the literature, but has been the subject of hardly any research. Usually, the absence of depression has been equated with denial (24). The psychological construct of denial is that reality in either a physical or emotional sense is subconsciously ignored or repressed by the individual. Denial is considered to be a maladaptive attempt to protect oneself from distress (25). Clinically, acute SCI patients are often observed to make statements that deny the reality of their injury, such as "When I'm walking again . . .", or "When I get back to my job unloading boxcars (or any other physically impossible occupation) . . . ." These statements and others do imply a sort of denial, but the truly important distinction is whether this denial is maladaptive.

Dr. Israel Goldiamond is another psychologist with a spinal cord injury. In his exploration of his own rehabilitation process (8), he points out:

> If I choose not to discuss my pains, problems, and infections, it is not because I am unaware, unrealistic, or repressing. At times I am painfully aware of them, and I mean that literally. If a patient does not face up to these issues, it may be because he is facing, or trying to face, in a different direction, one that can help him achieve his goals.

It seems that denial, as can depression, can serve a positive function for some individuals. By dealing with what is tolerable at that moment, the individual can keep from being overwhelmed and can continue to function appropriately. It seems quite rare that an individual who lives paralyzed for 24 hours a day is able to ignore that fact for a prolonged period of time. More common is the maintenance of a convenient fiction for a brief period during acute care in order to survive psychologically. There appears to be no need to ever force a newly injured SCI patient to "face reality."

PROGNOSIS

This chapter has presented the massive change that SCI brings, the hostile and unknown environment of acute care, the phsyical and psychological demands on the newly injured, and various commonly observed psychological reactions to this intense period. All of this is the necessary prelude to understanding the most crucial psychological event of this period—receiving one's prognosis, that one is paralyzed for life and there is no known cure.

Despite the inherently negative nature of SCI prognosis, the one study conducted on this subject found that 60% of a sample of 60 SCI patients felt that the ideal time to receive prognosis was within the first 2 weeks following injury. Another 25% of the sample felt that the timing depended on the individual, and only four patients felt that prognosis should be given later. Fully 87% of the sample felt that the physician should give the information to the patient. However, being told once is usually not enough.

Often during acute care, a patient returns to the question of prognosis with each of his or her caregivers. The question may be asked in a variety of ways, but its essence is always the same: "Will I walk again?" Every staff person involved in the acute care of a person with a SCI should be prepared for this question; yet, there is no one right answer.

There are, however, some useful, psychologically sound guidelines to follow in answering the question. First, the patient deserves an honest response. Trying to avoid the question only reduces the patient's confidence in the therapist. However, there are times when "I don't know" is an honest and truthful response. Second, respect and kindness are called for in this situation. No one needs to be told that such an important question is dumb or has already been answered several times. Third, hope is important for human beings and should be preserved. "I don't think so" is better than "no," and "It is very unlikely" is better than "never." Finally, as long as one is honest and clear there is no need to be right. If a patient needs to disagree with the staff, no harm is done. The information has been heard, and the patient will use it when it is tolerable to him or her.

FAMILY REACTION

The discussion of the acute phase of SCI has focused so far on the individual who is injured. However, the individual's family is also affected by the injury, is involved in acute care, and is influential in the adjustment process. Unfortunately, the health care system is primarily organized for care delivery to the identified patient. Families almost never receive as much professional attention as their loved one.

Some understanding of familial distress may enable allied health professionals to assist family members during the contacts that are made with them, however. The most visible family concerns are for the patient. Immediately following injury, the major problems relate to the communication of information. Due to the complexity of SCI a variety of medical specialties are generally involved in caring for the patient. One patient may be evaluated and treated by specialists in orthopedics, neurosurgery, neurology, radiology, general medicine, and rehabilitation medicine within 24 hr of admission. Each physician may speak to the family member about current findings and probable prognosis. The opportunities for communication problems are vast. Each specialist may have a different perspective and terminology that can be confusing to even the most sophisticated family member. Also, the patient's condition may be rapidly changing, so that yesterday's information is no longer valid and may even contradict today's data. Finally, different family members may be receiving different pieces of the whole picture and may communicate slight distortions to other family members so that the pieces no longer fit. Given these common problems in communication, it is not unusual for family members to become frustrated and distrustful of hospital personnel.

Emotionally, family members struggle with issues similar to those of the patient. They are also experiencing massive change, struggling with an unknown situation, and attempting to cope with the prognosis. In addition, family members often want to help but are not sure how, and they may be unsure about how to talk to their loved one. These feelings of helplessness, uncertainty, and distress may overlie unconscious feelings of guilt and/or anger related to the circumstances of the injury. It is not unusual for family members to experience poor sleep, decreased appetite, labile mood, and exacerbation of their own physical problems during this very difficult time.

Family members also have their own unique set of problems with which they must cope. These problems may include the mechanics of getting to the hospital, the reactions of children, coping with a sudden loss of income, dealing with insurance companies and lawyers, assuming an increase in household responsibilities, and perhaps taking over the family business. There is also the task of communicating with extended family and friends and attempting to absorb all of the various suggestions, advice, and information those people may offer.

Of course, all of this stress and strain occurs within the context of relationships that are established and have a history. Married couples may or may not have a strong and positive relationship. Parents may or may not feel good about the way their children have turned out. Children may or may not respect and admire their parents.

Clinical observation suggests that SCI does not change the nature of a particular relationship as much as it may magnify and intensify both its flaws and strengths. In the early phase of SCI, this "pressure cooker" effect is less apparent because of the almost overwhelming need for a variety of immediate responses. However, as a person with a SCI moves into the rehabilitation phase and the entire family begins to stabilize and plan for the future, these issues can loom very large.

PSYCHOLOGICAL INTERVENTION IN THE ACUTE CARE PHASE

What can rehabilitation professionals do to help patients and their families adjust psychologically to SCI during this acute phase of treatment? Unfortunately, there is no standard approach that can be used for every patient. Intervention must be tailored to the individual, the symptoms, and to the symptoms' underlying causes. Fortunately, a general understanding of what the patient and the family are experiencing can yield some general principles of intervention.

The first principle is to know the limitations of intervention. The acute care experience cannot be made a positive one, but its negatives can be reduced. All of the patient's and family's needs cannot be met by the rehabilitation team. Concentrating on meeting a smaller number of needs relevant to the rehabilitation process is much better than becoming overwhelmed by all the needs that one observes. Finally, it is important to remember that no able-bodied person can truly know what it is like to be paralyzed. Able-bodied individuals can definitely help, but to say "I know how you feel" is not a true statement and the patient knows this.

The second principle is to allow the patient to lead. By giving the patient the opportunity to talk and then listening carefully, the rehabilitation professional is in a position to actually know what concerns are important to the patient and to respond to those concerns. Good listening makes for efficient teaching and appropriate intervention. By allowing the patient to lead, his or her sense of control is also enhanced.

The third principle is to maintain the patient's dignity. In general, this means being polite and thoughtful. Specifically, it means drawing the curtain if the patient's body is going to be exposed. It means saying "please" and "thank you" to the patient. It also means addressing the patient formally—that is, Mr. or Ms.—until one receives permission to do otherwise. These relatively small details can afford the patient a sense of stability and adulthood in an otherwise unfamiliar and demeaning situation.

A fourth principle is to make the unknown known. This means teaching the patient about the new environment and its details. It means explaining treatments and their goals in terms the patient can readily understand. It means providing positive feedback for efforts that are adaptive and for any real progress that the patient makes. Yet, positive reinforcement is not particularly helpful if it is not attached to something meaningful. A patient who receives unconditional positive feedback has no greater understanding of the unknown than if he or she had received no feedback at all.

A fifth principle is to facilitate trust in the rehabilitation team. Trust can only be earned, but earning it is relatively simple: don't promise what you can't deliver, and make sure that what you do promise happens. If one promises to be there in the afternoon, be there. If one promises a procedure is not going to hurt, make sure it does not. If one promises to stop when the patient says stop, stop on command. By being reliable and trustworthy, the rehabilitation professional encourages the patient's trust. This ability to trust enables the patient to obtain the most out of the system at every point in time. We ask the patient and family to take much on faith; we must also demonstrate that their faith is well placed.

A final principle is always to strive to encourage positive, realistic expectancies. There is much that even the most severely injured person can accomplish. The rehabilitation professional must know and believe that fact. An attitude that a person is better off dead cannot be hidden, and anyone who feels that way should not work with SCI patients; these patients are too vulnerable. Of course there will be difficulties for the person with a SCI, but they are not insurmountable and they do not have to be overcome all at once. Patients who know this and who see this attitude in all around them have an adaptive start toward living with their injuries.

Rehabilitation Phase

The patient's experience of severe psychological crisis continues in the rehabilitation care setting. However, issues of life and death and physical safety are less prominent. Although all of the emotional reactions discussed earlier continue to be experienced by both the patient and the family, there is usually a degree of stability present by the time a patient is transferred to rehabilitation. Patients have begun to participate in their daily care programs. The potential for the permanent effects of injury has generally been absorbed by patient and family. They frequently have begun to perform the emotional balancing act of preparing for the worst and hoping for the best.

The rehabilitation phase of treatment is generally the most lengthy period of hospitalization following the initial injury. It is during this period that the patient and family begin the first steps toward eventual adjustment to the disability. These steps may be faltering and unsure, but they often set the pattern for the patient and family coping with the drastic changes brought on by SCI. It is during this period that most psychological intervention occurs and the patient's psychological gains will be conscious and remembered.

It is important to note that not every patient arrives at the rehabilitation setting having accomplished the psychological tasks described here under acute care. Occasionally, a patient arrives at rehabilitation with no understanding of the injury or prognosis or any foundation of knowledge to understand what has happened to him or her. These patients must spend the first period of time in rehabilitation dealing with the same types of issues and responses as described under acute care. However, for the majority of patients and their families the rehabilitation phase is initially a time for consolidation of gains and a time for psychological movement toward adaptive adjustment to their disability.

During this period, the patient should not be viewed or treated from the perspective of psychopathology. The exception to this rule would be those patients with a premorbid behavioral disturbance or maladaptive behavior pattern. Using the model of the psychopathology of behavior, the patients are assessed from the viewpoint of whether their actions represent an abnormal response to the normal events of everyday living. This is obviously an overly simplistic statement, but it is useful in pointing out an important difference in behavior observed after onset of the injury.

In contrast, the SCI patient's behavior represents a normal response to highly abnormal events: the stressful events of acute care and rehabilitation and the time following discharge as the patient attempts to resume life outside the hospital. These experiences are highly threatening. It is therefore necessary to view the patient's response and design intervention in the context of the psychology of crisis. In order to facilitate adaptive adjustment, psychological caregivers must have an understanding of the nature of adaptive adjustment.

THEORIES OF ADJUSTMENT

There are a number of reviews of theories of adjustment; yet, surprisingly few theories have been tested. However, a number of theories do have useful concepts that may be applied in various degrees in various cases. In clinical treatment, staff must be aware that patients present a wide variety of response styles, sources of primary distress, and approaches to restructuring a meaningful life. Although clearly defined or rigid structures pinpointing the steps along the way to adjustment may be helpful to staff in trying to comprehend the emotional experience of patients, these structures can be counterproductive if they are applied inflexibly. The importance of incorporating the role of individual differences in any theory of coping with SCI cannot be overemphasized.

A number of authors have described the rehabilitation program as a process of learning to live with disability within the environment. In discussing a model of psychological treatment during acute care following the onset of SCI, Meyerson's theory (10) has been reviewed. Significant elements of this theory include its definition of the process of rehabilitation and the specification of the procedures to accomplish rehabilitation. Rehabilitation is defined as learning how to interact with the environment to accomplish goals. Building a new repertoire of behavioral skills occurs through trial and error, training by successive approximation, or modeling. These processes should be performed more efficiently and more effectively in a formal rehabilitation unit.

Silver and Wortman (26) identify several models of adjustment to undesirable life events that offer different insights into the process of adjustment. Klinger suggests that a person's attention, thought content, and information processing are greatly influenced by the individually held goal incentive. Once blocked from achieving a desired goal, patients engage in cycles of incentive-disengagement with regard to goal attainment. Being blocked from attaining the goal leads first to an increased, vigorous focus upon the goal. When this attempt is thwarted, the response turns to anger, protest, and eventually to apathy and pessimism. Depression is seen as a normal part of disengagement from the goal. The incentive toward the goal lessens over time and is supposed to be replaced by pleasurable feelings directed to other goals.

Wortman and Brehm present a model of adjustment in which response invigoration or depression occurs, depending on the expectation of control over the outcome of the undesired event and the importance of the outcome. As the outcome is not controlled, depression and passivity are expected to result.

Seligman's model of learned helplessness is well known (27). The helpless response is seen as the outcome of how the patient (or subject) has interpreted an uncontrollable aversive stimulus. Interpretations or attributions are associated with maintenance of self-esteem and view the cause as stable and global. Those attributions directed toward the patient's own internal characteristics are associated with the loss of self-esteem.

Shontz proposes a series of stages to be passed through following a negative event or outcome (28). At the onset of a crisis, patients respond with anxiety and stress. During this period patterns of coping are not adequate. Shock as a reaction occurs as the inevitability of the undesired event becomes clear. Detachment and surprising efficiency of thought and action are also present. Next comes the encounter phase, with feelings of helplessness, panic, and disorganization. Problem-solving abilities may be impaired. A need to avoid the intensity of this period may cause some persons to "retreat," but only until they become aware of the inability to truly escape. Over time, cycles of encounter and retreat occur progressively less frequently. Each time a person begins a new phase of encountering reality, anxiety, frustration, and depression may occur. If these responses occur, they may be the precursors to positive psychological adjustment.

Lazarus presents several coping strategies that are equally important when the individual is faced with threats that become self-defined as a crisis (29). Rather than focusing simply on the coping styles of taking direct action, Lazarus presents inhibition of action, information seeking, and intrapsychic modes, such as thinking distracting or calming thoughts, as equally important approaches. The skills acquired through prior experiences and the ambiguity of the unmet crisis are likely determinants of which tactic is employed by the patient. One strength of Lazarus' formulation in applying to the process of coping with SCI is its emphasis on the importance of controlling or regulating one's own emotional state. Such control is essential if a patient is to be able to participate in the daily demands of a rehabilitation program, receive and comprehend the daily flood of information, and plan constructively for the numerous changes affecting his or her future.

A theory of cognitive adaptation described by Taylor has particular appeal (30). According to her formulation of the theory of cognitive adaptation, readjustment following a threatening event centers around three themes: a search for meaning, attempts to regain mastery over one's life, and efforts to enhance one's self-esteem.

Searching for meaning involves identifying why the event happened in one's life and assessing what impact the event has on one's life. In struggling to regain mastery over the event and one's life, the safety and the predictability of life are reconstructed. What needs to be done in order to prevent the future occurrence of this or other possibly related disasters is identified and attempted through action or alteration of one's personal belief system. Taylor proposes that all situations of victimization will lower self-esteem, regardless of the circumstances surrounding the event. Therefore, one major task of adjustment is the re-establishment of positive self-esteem. Social companions may play a major role in this process ("I am certainly better off than so and so").

Interestingly, Taylor contends that, as individuals face these three themes simultaneously, successful resolution depends on the ability to form and maintain a set of illusions. Events must become perceived from a different angle because analysis from formerly held positions or beliefs would lead to negative evaluations. ("I would be worthless if I could not do my construction job," or I would not want to live if I were permanently in a wheelchair.")

This concept is contrary to the traditional idea that positive mental health is based on being in touch with reality and not hiding behind illusions. However, it can easily be seen that the patient who persists in holding such former beliefs as being valued for physical prowess (as normally defined) or the importance of doing all activities just as they were done before injury is going to have a great deal of difficulty establishing a rewarding and meaningful life after discharge from the hospital. Illusion, or the alteration of one's belief system, is likely to serve a very beneficial protective role in the lives of SCI patients.

These theories of adjustment represent a selected sample of a larger number of available theories. Unfortunately, there exists no research showing that any one particular theory is the correct one to follow. Clinical experience suggests that the consistent application of a coherent theory generally helps the clinician proceed in an orderly manner toward facilitating the patient's adjustment. It is less a question of truth of a particular theory than a question of what helps the patient. A theoretical understanding of adjustment makes possible the variety of interventions that the psychologist and others utilize to help a person adjust to the massive change in his or her life known as SCI. In the following section, both general and specific interventions with patients are discussed.

PSYCHOLOGICAL INTERVENTION IN THE REHABILITATION PHASE

When faced with negative or devastating life events, most individuals benefit from having the opportunity to ventilate and simply talk about what is happening to them. Enabling the patient to talk about his or her concerns is one of the most basic but also most important roles the psychologist plays in the rehabilitation program. Therapeutic support can provide a positive setting that facilitates changes in the patient's own identity and increases self-confidence, as well as providing reinforcement for daily accomplishments. Taking time to hear regularly the details of the thoughts and emotional reactions of the patient can lessen the strain of the crisis and make it easier for the person to face the difficult task at hand.

During the rehabilitation phase, the psychologist expects to establish a strong relationship with the patient. Patients learn that generally speaking their level of distress is normal, not abnormal, and that no thought or feeling is forbidden or judged negatively. They understand that the psychologist expects to discuss any concern they have, even when other staff, family, or friends might be overwhelmed by their true feelings or thoughts or be too busy to listen. Patients also have the opportunity to test that any information that they want to be held in confidence will not be shared with the team or family. (The only exception to this principle of confidentiality is any information concerning a physical threat to anyone or any form of harm to children or vulnerable adults.)

These characteristics of the trusting and multifaceted relationship establish the foundation for accomplishing the tasks of behavior change that may be required in the later stages of psychological rehabilitation.

Within the body of psychological literature, there is an area of research that describes characteristics of the population who benefit from psychotherapy (31). This group is generally described as bright, verbal, and from middle and upper socioeconomic backgrounds. Interestingly enough, the authors have found that in clinical practice with spinal cord injured patients active participation in psychotherapy occurs in the majority of cases. Many patients who would not be described as psychologically insightful and verbal by traditional psychological measures respond positively to psychotherapeutic interventions. It is possible that the distress of the crisis state following injury allows receptivity to self-exploration and malleability of behavior patterns in individuals who would generally not respond to psychological intervention techniques.

Individual Therapy. Individual therapy forms the basic foundation for psychological intervention with SCI patients in the rehabilitation setting. These individual contacts may be formal sessions behind closed doors or more frequent informal contacts on the ward itself. As the patient's medical stability increases. his or her independence begins to increase and daily life becomes more predictable and secure. As a result, the true individuality of each patient's personality is expressed more clearly in a hospital setting. The person's own pattern of psychological and behavioral strengths and weaknesses is more evident. The nature of the patient's interpersonal relationships also becomes clearer.

Individual therapy also uncovers the individual's premorbid skills and characteristics, such as the ability to tolerate frustration, to solve problems, to rally support and resources, to create cooperation among those around them, to set goals and to plan strategies to achieve those goals, and to have confidence in being able to influence the course of life. This knowledge enables patients to make the most of their strengths and to identify and compensate for their areas of weakness.

It should be remembered that generally speaking many of the behavioral skill deficits common among SCI patients seem to be a function of the youthfulness of this population, rather than a form of psychopathology. Many skills that are adaptive in a crisis are usually acquired in young adulthood and maturity as part of the normal human developmental process (32). Therefore, it is important to keep in mind the base rates of the occurrence of these skills in the peer age group of each patient. In many respects, successful progress in rehabilitation demands higher-level behavioral skills than does normal activity in the community. The ability of the majority of patients to meet these challenges successfully warrants the recognition and respect of rehabilitation professionals.

Family Therapy. Another type of psychological intervention used to facilitate adjustment is family therapy. Just as the true complexity of each patient's individual personality style and behavioral patterns becomes clearer in individual therapy, the nature of the status of premorbid relationships in the patient's life generally becomes more evident during family therapy.

It is not uncommon for long-standing conflicts at home to emerge while the person is hospitalized. For instance, parents may have repeatedly argued about a child's speeding while driving and being in accidents or in legal trouble in the past. Perhaps the child was planning to move away or had recently moved away from home when the SCI occurred. Even though all members of the family may want desperately for everything to be done for the injured family member, they may have strong doubts and fears about the child returning to the home after discharge. In this situation, the difficult task of family therapy is to negotiate a tolerable form of conflict resolution and mutual respect. In the event that no resolution is possible, the psychologist may need to inform the rehabilitation team that a return to the home environment is likely to be detrimental to the patient and that other living arrangements need to be investigated.

Previous patterns of conflict in marriages are also often revealed in the rehabilitation setting. A marriage with a history of imbalance in dominance or dependence or with a pattern of unresolved long-standing conflict is often unable to adapt quickly or at all to the additional stress of SCI. As the patient and spouse in couple's therapy become able to examine their feelings or concerns together, while learning nonthreatening communication skills perhaps for the first time, plans for the future can be developed.

In contrast, when a patient and spouse have a history of working as a team, have a nonavoidant and nonconfrontational style of sharing distress, and have successfully adapted to unwanted circumstances in the past, there is a different role for intervention. Here, frequent support and education from staff can assist the couple in resuming a pattern of cooperation in attaining shared goals and reaffirming mutual respect.

Effect of Prior Emotional Trauma. In clinical practice, the authors have frequently encountered a significant psychological response to injury that is generally not discussed in the rehabilitation literature. Following injury, a patient's current emotional distress may reinstate or reawaken an experience of emotional trauma from the individual's past. Therefore, in addition to the extreme distress that frequently accompanies the beginning of life with a SCI, the individual must also cope with reliving elements of the anxiety of an earlier trauma or state of extended crisis. Individuals who may be particularly vulnerable to the additional emotional upheaval are those whose histories include individual traumatic events or who have lived through periods of stress or trauma.

Examples of the experiences of individual traumatic events are patients with histories of child abuse, rape, other criminal victimization, or the death of loved ones. Patients who have lived through extended periods of childhood abuse, military service during war, and incarceration in prison may also relive the earlier trauma. The emotions highlighted by these memories include fear, panic, hopelessness, anger, and complete loss of control over one's life. In some cases, the patient may become so overwhelmed by reliving the past emotional trauma that he or she does not experience the immediate distress of the onset of injury. The psychologist must address the need of the patient for restored safety and emotional security through either individual or family therapy. As soon as this can be accomplished, therapy can be directed toward the issues of self-exploration and education about learning to manage psychologically as a person with a SCI.

Group Therapy. Another very powerful form of intervention to facilitate adjustment to disability is group psychotherapy. In recent years, therapeutic groups for rehabilitation patients have become more and more popular. The reason for this popularity lies in the inherent positive power of a group of SCI patients sharing together, identifying together, and helping one another along this most difficult of paths toward adjustment.

Groups not only provide significant opportunities for self-exploration and greater understanding of one's relationship with others but they also help reduce one's sense of isolation and foster a sense of power and control. Although a SCI group session may be intense and painful, it is often also raucous and enjoyable. Many times this wide variety of group interactions can provide benefits to the patient that no interaction with an able-bodied person can. SCI groups demonstrate the truth of the old cliche that there is strength in numbers.

Vocational Evaluation. One final type of intervention a psychologist may use to foster an adaptive adjustment toward disability and an optimistic orientation toward the future is to initiate an educational/vocational evaluation. Such evaluations may involve the use of objective psychological instruments to establish vocational interest, aptitude, and readiness. Even if the patient is not ready to make decisions about his or her future role in the world of work, beginning an evaluation can establish the positive expectation that an active work role can be created. Once this expectation is established, it can be nurtured and can gradually come to full fruition. Even if only the stage of brainstorming of ideas about a future work role is achieved, it can have a positive therapeutic effect with SCI patients.

PSYCHOSOCIAL ISSUES THAT MAY IMPEDE PROGRESS

Psychological interventions perform a variety of functions during the rehabilitation program, including alleviation of extreme anxiety, fear, and panic; providing relief from overwhelming distress elicited by reliving past trauma, identifying behavioral repertoire deficits; teaching adaptive patterns of response; and influencing a positive restructuring of self-image as the meaning of the injury and its impact on life are explored by each patient.

Several factors may impede progress in rehabilitation. The importance of having a variety of behavioral skills to assist in coping with life with an unwanted disability has already been mentioned. The ability to behave in a way that fosters the cooperation and support of others will serve the patient well in achieving goals throughout his or her life. Many patients must learn the skill of assessing a problem situation, identifying a means of solving the problem, and persisting in behavior over time to achieve the solution goal. Most people must also master a strategy for structuring day-to-day activities to provide positive and meaningful experiences that enhance the development of a meaningful life, positive self-image, and feelings of self-worth.

Another factor that may limit or slow progress in long-term adaptation to SCI is an inadequate social support system. Polletts (13) found that, in addition to medical and socioeconomic variables, perceived social support was an important factor in adjustment of his sample of SCI patients. Therefore, an important skill to be taught to each patient by the psychologist and others is the ability to assess the available support network. These skills will be important following discharge and can benefit the patient throughout his or her life.

Sexuality. A factor that is usually not thought of as a psychological adjustment factor, but which is extremely important to the individual patient and his or her family, is sexuality. SCI affects human sexuality in a large number of ways from both a purely physical and a purely psychological standpoint. The literature on SCI is filled with articles on sexuality. In many ways, the SCI population has been the model for developing materials and intervention strategies on human sexuality for rehabilitation patients. This is fortunate, given the importance of sexuality to this rather young and aggressive group of rehabilitation patients. The information in this chapter does not attempt to make the reader an expert on human sexuality. For that, the reader should pursue some of the very excellent and extensive materials that are already available to the allied health professional. This section does provide an overview for the person who is planning to work with spinal cord injured persons, however.

Psychologically, sexuality can be construed as an extremely broad and basic part of each individual's personality. From earliest childhood, each of us identifies ourselves as either male or female, and the basis for this identification is clearly our sexuality. It is an understatement to say that in American culture this sexual identification is pervasive and important.

Spinal cord injury can force individuals to re-examine lifelong assumptions about their own identity and their place in our culture and world. Whether the SCI individual is involved in individual, family, or group therapy while in rehabilitation, no therapeutic endeavor should fail to include these issues at several points in time throughout rehabilitation. However, the patient's interest and concerns in sexuality are rarely limited to these types of formal interventions. Every member of the SCI treatment team will experience the patient's exploration of sexuality following SCI to some extent.

On the physical level, SCI may cause a wide range of changes in sexual function and expression. These changes are exceedingly complex and are dependent upon the patient's level of injury, completeness of injury, and gender. For an injured male, physical change may include alterations in erections, sensation, ejaculation, fertility, and orgasmic response. The nerve roots that control these sexual functions are closely related to the nerve paths that control bladder and bowel function; therefore bowel and bladder function will often provide the first clues as to the injured individual's ultimate sexual function. At one end of the spectrum, a complete, cervical level injury may probably result in the individual being able to experience a reflex erection with no sensation, impaired ejaculatory response, and low fertility. However, there is increasing evidence of a relearned orgasmic response to alternative stimulation for these individuals, as well as considerable evidence of an active sexual existence for even high-level quadriplegics. At the other end of the spectrum, a low-level injury that allows for an individual to have normal bowel and bladder function may well result in minimal physical changes in sexual response. Between these two extremes almost any pattern of sexual response changes can be found. Perhaps the most important fact for the patient to know is that, no matter what the pattern of sexual changes is because of the SCI, an active and rewarding sexual existence is possible. This is a reality that has been demonstrated many times by many patients. There appears to be very little that is automatic about a healthy sexual adjustment to SCI, however, and it almost always requires considerable communication between partners and an active desire to explore and rebuild a sexual relationship.

For females, sexual changes are as variable and as crucial as for males. However, the pattern of physical changes is different. Although a woman may experience similar changes in sensation, organic orgasmic response, and physical limitations in the sexual act, the reproductive changes caused by SCI are generally less severe for the female than for the male. For the most part, spinal cord injured women are able to conceive, carry to term, and deliver normal and healthy children. However, women carry a somewhat different burden because of the norms of contemporary American culture. Our culture places such a high value on attractiveness for women that the spinal cord injured female may often be devastated by feelings of diminished attractiveness and limitations in her abilities to give and receive affection physically.

For both male and female spinal cord injured patients, the rehabilitation phase often provides the first opportunity for them to explore and redefine their sense of personal sexuality. Often this process is both verbal and behavioral, and it may involve a variety of members of the SCI treatment team. Generally, the patient addresses these issues with those staff members whom he or she trusts and admires the most. For this reason, every member of the SCI treatment team must be prepared to address issues of sexuality to some extent when the patient raises them. However, in this area, as in most others that have been discussed, patient variability is extremely large, and there is no one correct way of dealing with every patient's concerns.

Sexual concerns may be expressed overtly and directly, they may be expressed in subtle and oblique ways, or they may be acted out in public and potentially embarrassing ways. Of course, some patients may never express them at all.

The question then becomes what can the allied health profession do to facilitate a healthy sexual readjustment on the part of the spinal cord injured patient. Although there is no standard approach to every patient's sexual concerns, there are a number of actions that allied health professionals can take to prepare themselves in this area. Any rehabilitation professional who wishes to make SCI his or her area of professional expertise needs to do three things in order to address adequately patient's concerns about sexuality. First, the professional needs to have an honest and thorough understanding of his or her own personal sexuality. This self-knowledge includes an understanding of one's own sexual values, biases, and problem areas. Every human being has limits to his or her own sexuality. As professionals, we must know our own limits so that we do not impose them upon our patients.

The second action that a health care professional must take in preparation is to acquire knowledge about human sexuality in general and SCI sexuality in particular. One needs to understand anatomy and physiology, the sexual response cycle, and the range of human sexual behavior in our culture. This information can be found in current textbooks on human sexuality and the professional literature on SCI. This factual information provides the foundation for understanding and being able to explain the changes in human sexuality brought on by SCI. Although not all of the patient's concerns about sexuality are questions that can be answered by factual information, questions of fact are often the starting point for sexual adjustment. Possessing factual knowledge provides credibility to the health care professional.

Experience in dealing with this area is the third important factor in facilitating sexual adjustment. Although there is no true substitute for the hands-on experience of dealing with patients, one can plan ahead by talking to more experienced staff members so that one may be better prepared when the issue of sexuality is raised. Even though sexuality is an area of extreme sensitivity and confidentiality, staff members need to be able to share their own reactions and responses in order to ensure that the patient's needs are being met. An excellent list of guidelines for dealing with sexual issues in spinal cord injury is found in the work of Dr. George Hohmann (15). It is highly recommended that any professional who will be working with SCI patients read extensively in the area of human sexuality, as well as consult with more experienced professionals.

Alcohol and Drug Abuse. A final factor that may impede progress in rehabilitation is a pattern of alcohol and drug use. There is considerable evidence that SCI patients as a group have higher intake patterns than the population as a whole.

Sweeney and Foote (33) noted that many injuries occur as a result of a drug or alcohol use life-style. In this study, injuries were frequently associated with chemical intake and violence. Redd (34) found that 11.4% of a sample of 35 SCI patients had ingested one to two alcoholic beverages within 2 hr of becoming injured. An additional 34.3% had taken three or more alcoholic drinks within 2 hr of being injured. In this study an empirically derived personality scale designed to measure a characteristic of enduring vulnerability to excessive alcohol use also suggests that these patients were at high risk (35). The group mean score on this scale was not significantly different from the problem drinker (DWI) norm group. Adair, Heinemann, Donohue, and Goddard (36) reported that 47% of a sample of 47 SCI patients were under the influence of alcohol or drugs at the time of injury. These patients also reported significantly more adverse effects from substance use before they became spinal cord injured.

Rehabilitation programs for SCI patients need to address substance abuse issues directly because these patients are at risk for substance abuse after discharge from rehabilitation. These patients may lack alternatives to creating feelings of exhilaration and experiencing a release from tension and frustration. They are often ill-prepared for coping with the stress of re-entering the world as a disabled person. They often have an established preinjury pattern of heavy use. Physicians often prescribe medications that may lead to addiction. The combination of prescribed medications with over-the-counter and recreational drugs and alcohol can be very dangerous. In addition, drinking and drug taking may be one of the few social activities that patients can still participate in as easily as they could before being injured. Patients may adopt chemical use as a means of tolerating a life-style characterized by inactivity, boredom, and isolation.

It is important to design educational and psychotherapeutic interventions in rehabilitation settings for both patient and family members to encourage lowered chemical use or abstinence. Many SCI rehabilitation programs will be offering these services in the near future. It is hoped that outcome studies will be available in the near future.

THERAPEUTIC RECREATION

In all model SCI treatment centers and a growing number of general hospitals and rehabilitation centers, recreational therapy has become an increasingly important therapeutic activity for spinal cord injured patients. Due in large part to Guttmann in England, there exists a large body of literature demonstrating the efficacy of sports and leisure activities as therapeutic endeavors (37).

Clinically, the authors have observed that recreational activities provide opportunities for newly injured individuals to expand their behavioral repertoire in a nonthreatening manner and to reassert themselves as active, competitive individuals. Therapeutic recreation spans the entire range of leisure activities. Spinal cord injured individuals participate in competitive athletics (basketball, football, track and field, marathons, swimming, bowling, archery, weight lifting, etc.); individual recreational pursuits (sailing, scuba diving, flying, snow skiing, auto racing, hunting, fishing, etc.); and social activities (shopping, dancing, camping, travel, etc.). Leisure activities are limited only by the person's inclination and imagination. There seems to be little doubt that an active recreational therapy program can greatly facilitate long-term adjustment to disability for spinal cord injured individuals.

DISCHARGE PLANNING

The final phase of rehabilitation is preparation for discharge, although discharge planning actually takes place throughout the hospitalization. Generally, discharge planning is the sum total of efforts specifically aimed at planning and problem solving for the individual's return to his or her home environment. It includes, but is not limited to, trial home passes, evaluating the home environment for adaptive modifications, establishing a vocational plan, obtaining adaptive equipment and aids if required, and, often, driver's training. Depending upon the needs of the individual, discharge planning services may include all of these aspects, a smaller number, or an even larger number.

Discharge planning is primarily focused on transferring the individual from the rehabilitation environment to the home environment with the least amount of dislocation possible. By considering and solving as many problems as possible before discharge, the inherent trauma of resuming living in the everyday world is reduced as much as possible. However, it has been observed that the period immediately following the rehabilitation phase is one of the most trying and difficult times for the newly injured person with a SCI.

After Discharge

Following discharge from rehabilitation, the spinal cord injured person faces perhaps the greatest challenge of all—living as a disabled person for the rest of his or her life. Success at this formidable task is difficult to define and measure. What is successful for one person might be intolerable for another, and no single measure can be used to evaluate outcome. Perhaps the best we can do is to consider the results of rehabilitation efforts in terms of adaptiveness. Three areas of adaptiveness seem to be most important: maintaining health and avoiding the preventable complications of SCI; leading an active, productive life; and finally, achieving an appropriate degree of life satisfaction. In psychological terms, these three forms of adapting can be viewed as caring enough about oneself to protect one's health consistently; to be involved in the larger world in a contributory manner; and to feel satisfied about one's sense of self, one's relationships, and one's accomplishments.

Of course, psychological factors are not the only determinants of life with a SCI. For any individual living life with a disability, psychological factors are intertwined through all phases of one's life, and they both influence and are influenced by one's skills, strengths, weaknesses, circumstances, friends, family, opportunities, and culture. The following section surveys the common issues a spinal cord injured person may face following rehabilitation, with an emphasis on the role of psychology in these issues. As with all things psychological, generalizations tend to be dangerously misleading. Each person with a spinal cord injury is a unique individual and will approach his or her life after rehabilitation in unique ways.

Perhaps the first problem many former spinal cord patients face when returning home is a total lack of structure to their lives. For months they existed in a hospital setting where they were told what to do, when to do it, and how to do it. One's home, the object of desire for all those months in the hospital, is different and difficult. There may be no reason to get up in the morning at any particular time, and in some cases, getting up early in the morning may even put an extra burden on an already overburdened spouse. There is no set schedule of events, and some people find filling their time a difficult task. It is the rare person who leaves the hospital and immediately re-enters the work world and his or her own personal activities of daily living.

In addition, activities may seem harder to do at home. All the various skills, so painfully acquired in the hospital, may be difficult to apply to the home environment. Shag carpets may be substituted for tile floors, narrow hallways for wide corridors, and small rooms for large ones. There is often a strong desire to let someone else do things for one because it is so much easier.

Weekend passes were helpful in reducing the strangeness of home and anticipating many of the concrete problems, but a person soon learns that a 2-day break from the hospital is not the same as actually living at home. For the spouse, the rest period when the injured person returned to the hospital is no longer available, and there is a great deal to do everyday. For many spouses, not only is there a lot to do, but it all has to be done correctly or there could be dire consequences. For the former patient, there is no longer an army of experienced nurses available around the clock, and what happens if something goes wrong? There are no longer doctors on call or even call lights to summon assistance. Even if these emergency measures have not been actually needed for some time, for many people the absence of these symbols of security awakens some of the same fears experienced soon after the injury. In some ways it is ironic that, once personal control again becomes possible for the individual, it may be accompanied by feelings of helplessness and dependency.

Although there is little formal research on this period of adjustment to the home environment, it has been clinically observed that most former patients and their families somehow muddle through this time. Some people simply "fly through it" and do exceptionally well. Others struggle for many months. The basic psychological issue seems to be one of role redefinition. The injury itself has stripped the individual of many of his or her personal roles, such as adult, worker, spouse, and parent; leaving the hospital has stripped the individual of those roles that were supplied in the aftermath of the injury, such as physical therapy patient, occupational therapy patient, and nursing problem. Returning home but being still unable to resume all of the old roles leaves the person in a type of psychological limbo.

What is needed is for the individual to be able to define him- or herself in relation to family, friends, and the world at large. This definition of self is a highly variable and complex activity. It actually involves many roles in many different situations, and the individual needs to re-explore all of the old roles to see which ones still fit, as well as develop new roles. Nothing is static about this process. Development ranges across a wide variety of situations and varies considerably with time and the aging process.

BASIC ADJUSTMENTS

The most basic adjustments often come first. The newly discharged individual needs to learn how to get around in his or her own home: transferring in and out of bed, getting dressed, maneuvering the wheelchair around the home, and perhaps fixing meals or doing other chores around the house. All of these basic mobility issues need to be resolved as soon as possible, and the amount of difficulties the person faces in resolving them should not be underestimated. Unlike rehabilitation centers, American homes are not designed for people who rely on wheelchairs. A slight difference in the height of the bed, the difference in closets, the differences in the kitchen, the differences in the hallways of the house all can make previously learned behaviors more difficult or even inappropriate. Too many times, housing modifications are incomplete at the time of discharge, or perhaps there is no money available to modify the house at all. Yet, if the individual cannot move around in his or her own house or get in and out of the house, he or she will be unable to interact with the rest of the world in any meaningful or regular way. Of course, for those who are able to negotiate this first stumbling block, it turns out to be only the first of many hurdles.

Once a person can move around the home and get in and out of the house, the problem of transportation must then be faced. For some people, resolving this problem is as simple as putting an inexpensive set of hand controls into an already owned automobile. For others, transportation involves the purchase and modification of new vehicles. For others, transportation involves hiring someone to do the transporting. And for still others, transportation involves attempting to use public means of transportation, usually a difficult and frustrating task. However, without transportation an individual is virtually a prisoner in his or her own home.

Once an individual has solved the problem of basic, reliable transportation, there then exists the larger problem of accessibility. An individual may be able to get out and to travel, but getting into the destination involves an entirely new set of barriers. Is there parking? Are there steps? Are there elevators? Are there bathrooms? These questions and more must be faced each time a new place is confronted. Once one's own community is successfully mapped out and negotiated, there still remains the larger world. Traveling long distances brings its own challenges and demands. Is the plane accessible? Is the hotel accessible? Is camping possible? Is overseas travel still possible? What if . . .?

Mobility, transportation, accessibility, and travel represent extremely important but extremely basic issues. Obviously they can be solved because they have been solved by others, but the solutions are often not clear. In order for people to master their environment, they need to be able to adopt the roles of a determined person, a creative person, and an expert problem solver. In addition to these personal resources, they also need financial resources and considerable family and community support. However, solving these basic problems cannot be a full-time job, for there are a number of other roles that the person with a SCI must explore, develop, and master.

SOCIAL ADJUSTMENT

Socially, the individual must start with adjustments to the most immediate family and gradually move outward again. If the person is married, the issues of resuming the spousal role are extremely important. Differentiating between the person's spouse as caregiver and lover can sometimes be a difficult task. The very nature of a previously developed marital relationship may have to be completely reworked. Sometimes the injured individual is unable to physically resume previous roles. Sometimes the noninjured partner has had to learn new roles and has grown into a new understanding of him- or herself and the role in the relationship. It is probably a testament to the strength of the human spirit and the resiliency of the human character that the divorce rate among couples where one partner has received a SCI is no higher than the national average (5).

Children in a marriage raise another whole set of social issues. An individual needs to relearn the role of parent. Previously enjoyed activities may need to be modified or occasionally abandoned. The means of discipline may need to be changed, and the whole role of authority in relation to children may need to be re-examined. Often, children have many questions about their parent's new status and necessary routines. Occasionally, a parent is in the home for a longer time than he or she used to be, thereby causing new types of conflicts to emerge. Fortunately, research again fails to demonstrate any systematic harm to children as the result of having a disabled parent (38, 39).

For unmarried individuals, the issues of courtship often loom large. Believing oneself to be attractive and desirable is often a major concern for the spinal cord injured individual and has been cited as a primary concern by many females with a SCI (20). Achieving intimacy with an able-bodied person requires the ability to break through social barriers and stereotypes (40). Fortunately, there are many examples of successful courtships and sound and successful marriages among individuals with a spinal cord injury (5). In fact, the divorce rate for those persons who marry after their injury is considerably lower than the national average (5). However, the statistics also demonstrate that fewer disabled people get married than is the national norm (41). Courtship is clearly difficult, although it is not an impossible task.

Summary

Psychological adjustment to SCI is a complex and often painful process. Although certain broad generalities can be cited concerning the personalities of many people who suffer a SCI, their early experiences in acute care setting, and tasks they must accomplish during and following rehabilitation, every spinal cord injured person is truly unique. They bring their own learning history to their injury and attempt to do the best they can to adapt to a sudden, negative change in almost every phase of their life. Psychologists and other allied health professionals do their best to facilitate adjustment to disability, but this seldom represents the entire story of adjustment. Individuals use their own inner resources, the strength and support they find from their family and friends, and the encouragement and honesty of other patients in order to maximize the quality of their life following this devastating injury. It truly is a testament to basic human strength and flexibility that so many patients do so well. We have found that the opportunity to participate in this remarkable process is what makes the challenge, hard work, and emotional distress of working with spinal cord injured patients worthwhile.

Beyond the family there exists the individual's network of friends and acquaintances. Most individuals with SCI are able to tell of close friends who are unable to continue the friendship following their injury. Some able-bodied individuals are extremely uncomfortable with disabled people and for a multitude of reasons are unable to tolerate their presence. Other friends are lost when activities and recreational pursuits are no longer mutually shared. However, other friendships are deepened and strengthened by the adversity of SCI. Communication and sharing seem to reach new and deeper levels. New activities and interests also bring new friendships and social contacts.

The importance of family and friends cannot be overestimated. Recent research into perceived social support suggests that an individual's social network plays an extremely important part in the overall adaptation to living with a SCI (13). It is probable that, for most of us, the way that we perceive ourselves affects how others treat us. Of course, family and friends do not represent the entire story of adapting socially. There always remains that larger body pf people known as the "public."

For many spinal cord injured individuals, dealing with the public is a never-ending chore. People's curiosity about people in wheelchairs, who are a fairly uncommon sight, is fairly understandable. Heads turn and individuals look, and often curiosity leads them to ask questions. While any one individual looking and asking is a rather minor annoyance at worst, this phenomenon tends to grow irritating with time. The spinal cord injured person must learn to deal with a never-ending stream of people looking and asking questions. In addition, people often fail to notice the individual who is below their line of sight, which may make negotiating public spaces a trying and frustrating experience.

Unfortunately, being visibly different also attracts those who have their own personal difficulties. Although rare, interactions that are belligerent, hostile, or bigoted do occur, and people in wheelchairs can sometimes be viewed as easy prey for the psychopathic, criminal element among us. Fortunately much more common, although sometimes as irritating, is the overly helpful individual: the person who wants to help by grabbing the wheelchair and pushing, offering helpful advice, or just trying to do good. Helpful and harmful, curious and oblivious, ignorant and arrogant, the spinal cord injured individual must learn to deal with them all if he or she is to function among the public places of our culture.

Adapting to the physical and social environment is an extremely demanding task for the spinal cord injured individual. It requires a great deal of energy, skill, and fortitude. It is little wonder that some authors have suggested that a person with a SCI should not even consider work for a year or 2 years or even longer following injury. It is also understandable that at least one nationwide study of psychological reaction to SCI found that the maximum amount of psychological distress does not occur in the first month after injury or even the first year after injury, but occurs approximately 3–5 years following injury when the person has finally felt the total impact of SCI upon his or her life (W Dexter, personal communication). One study also suggests that this is the period when the spinal cord injured individual is most at risk for committing suicide (42).

A more common danger appears to be what Ernst Bors called "psychological suicide" (43). These are the cases where individuals' distress leads them to neglect their physical well-being or to indulge in such practices as drug and alcohol abuse that are extremely harmful in the long run. Fortunately, the number of people with SCI who are seriously harmed by this psychological distress seems to be relatively small. Far more individuals appear to engage in active and productive lives.

For many years, the sole criterion for successful rehabilitation following SCI was a return to productive work. Most spinal cord injured patients were rehabilitated under the auspices of their state vocational rehabilitation agencies, and those agencies were primarily concerned with competitive employment and/or enrollment in formal educational programs. The literature on vocational outcome contains many studies measuring these factors. However, this simplistic approach to outcome tended to yield rather disappointing results. Various authors cited return to work statistics ranging from 13% (44) to around 50% (7, 45). Occasionally, some studies would yield somewhat higher return to work statistics. But, in general, the statistics of re-employment were somewhat disappointing.

There are a number of reasons why spinal cord injured people do not return to competitive employment. Two of the most common barriers to employment help reveal why this single-minded approach to measuring outcome is less than ideal. First, there are the financial disincentives to resuming work. Many people with spinal cord injuries receive some type of disability benefits as a result of their injuries. Often, these financial resources, although limited, are extremely important to the survival of the individual. A person who resumes work may lose all of these benefits. Generally, it is not the funds per se that act as the disincentive. Rather, the individual becomes ineligible for various forms of service that are extremely expensive to procure privately. These services may include medical care, attendant care, and the equipment and supplies necessary for survival as a spinal cord injured person. When a person returns to work and is forced to purchase these necessary items, the financial burden is staggering. No entry-level job can provide a salary adequate to cover these needs. This tends to discourage many people from resuming competitive employment at anything less than the very top levels of the job market (46).

A second barrier to resuming competitive employment lies in the reluctance of employers to hire spinal cord injured persons. Many surveys and research projects have demonstrated a continuing reluctance on the part of employers to take the perceived risks involved in hiring a person in a wheelchair. Often-cited concerns by employers include the need for building modifications, insurance risks, and fears for their company's public image (47). Although great strides have been made in these areas through both educational and legislative efforts, it remains difficult for the spinal cord injured individual to find employers who are willing to take these perceived risks. Thus, we can begin to see why factors external to the individual and the rehabilitation he or she has received can influence return to competitive employment.

A more fruitful look at outcome is characterized by studies that measure a wider range of behaviors that can be grouped together as productivity measures. Productivity includes not only competitive employment but also sheltered employment, volunteer services, home-making activities, and community service. This approach to measuring outcome also usually includes the individual's involvement in avocational pursuits. These types of studies generally tend to suggest a much higher rate of return to productivity (6).

References

1. Woodbury B, Ditunno JF: Acute psychosis in traumatic spinal cord injury. Presented at the American Spinal Injury Association, Denver, 1983.
2. Trieschmann R: *Spinal Cord Injuries: The Psychological, Social, and Vocational Adjustment*. Elmsford, NY, Pergamon Press, 1980.
3. Crewe N, Krause J: Psychological aspects of spinal cord injury. In Caplan B (ed): *Rehabilitation Psychology Desk Reference*. Rockville, MD, Aspen Publishers, 1987.
4. Fordyce WE: Behavioral methods in rehabilitation. In Neff WS (ed): *Rehabilitation Psychology*. Washington, DC, American Psychological Association, 1971, pp 74–108.
5. El Ghatit A, Hanson R: Outcome of marriages existing at the time of a male's spinal

cord injury. *J Chron Dis* 28:383–388, 1975.

6. Kemp B, Vash C: Productivity after injury in a sample of spinal cord injured persons: A pilot study. *J Chron Dis* 24:259–275, 1971.

7. Brown B, Chanin I: Patterns of education and employment: Rehabilitants from severe spinal cord injury. *Rehabil Res Rep* 30:1972–73, 1974.

8. Goldiamond I: A diary of self-modification. *Psychology Today* 7:95–100, November, 1973.

9. Mosak H: Performance of the Harrower-Erikson multiple choice test of patients with spinal cord injuries. *J Consult Clin Psychol* 15:346–249, 1951

10. Meyerson L: Somatopsychology of physical disability. In Cruickshank WM (ed): *Psychology of Exceptional Children and Youth*, ed 3. Englewood Cliffs, NJ, Prentice-Hall, 1971, pp 1–74.

11. Lewin K: *The Conceptual Representation and the Measurement of Psychological Forces*. Durham, NC, Duke University Press, 1938.

12. Roberts A: Spinal Cord Injury; Some psychological considerations. *Minn Med* 55:1115–1117, 1972.

13. Polletts D: *The relationship between perceived social support and outcome following spinal cord injury*. Presented at the annual meeting of the Am Congress of Rehab Med, Kansas City, 1985.

14. Kerr W, Thompson M: Acceptance of disability of sudden onset in paraplegia. *Int J Paraplegia* 10:94–102, 1972.

15. Hohmann G: Psychological aspects of treatment and rehabilitation of the spinal injured person. *Clin Orthop* 112:81–88, 1975.

16. Caywood TA: A quadriplegic young man looks at treatment. *J Rehabil* 49:22–25, 1974.

17. Siller J: Psychological situation of the disabled with spinal cord injuries. *Rehabil Lit* 30:290–296, 1969.

18. Bourstrom NC, Howard MT: Personality characteristics of three disability groups. *Arch Phys Med Rehabil* 46:626–632, 1965.

19. Lawson N: *Depression after spinal cord injury: A multi-level longitudinal approach*. Ph.d. Dissertation, University of Houston, 1976.

20. Deyoe F: Marriage and family patterns with long-term spinal cord injury. *Int J Paraplegia* 10:219–224, 1972.

21. Kalb M: *An examination of the relationship between hospital ward behaviors and post-discharge behaviors in the spinal cord injury patients*. Ph.D. dissertation, University of Houston, 1971.

22. Seligman M: *Helplessness: On depression, Development and Death*. San Francisco, WH Freeman, 1975.

23. Costello C: Depression: Loss of reinforcers or loss of reinforcer effectiveness? *Behav Ther* 3:240–247, 1972.

24. Dembo T, Leviton G, Wright B: Adjustment to misfortune—a problem of social-psychological rehabilitation. *Rehabil Psychol* 22:1–100, 1975.

25. Bernstein L, Bernstein R: *Interviewing: A Guide for Health Professionals*, ed 3 New York, Appleton-Century-Crofts, 1980.

26. Silver R, Wortman CB: Coping with undesirable life events. In Garber J, Seligman M (eds): *Human Helplessness: Theory and Applications*. New York, Academic Press, 1980, pp 279–340.

27. Wortman CB, Brehm JW: Responses to uncontrollable outcomes; An integration of reactance theory and the learned helplessness model. In Berkowitz L (ed): *Advances in Experimental Social Psychology*. New York, Academic Press, 1975, Vol 8.

28. Shontz FC: Physical disability and personality: Theory and recent research. *Psychol Aspects Disability* 17:51–69, 1970.

29. Lazarus A: Learning theory and the treatment of depression. *Behav Res Ther* 6:83–89, 1968.

30. Taylor SE: Adjustment to threatening events. *Am Psychologist* 38:1161–1172, 1983.

31. Garfield SL: Research on client variables in psychotherapy. In Bergin AE, Garfield SL (eds): *Handbook of Psychotherapy and Behavior Change*. New York, John Wiley & Sons, 1974, pp 271–298.

32. Devnetsky J: *Psychology*. San Francisco, West Publishing Co, 1985.

33. Sweeney FF, Foote JE: Treatment of drug and alcohol abuse in spinal cord injured veterans. *Inter J Addictions* 17:897–904, 1982.

34. Redd CL: *Vulnerability to alcohol abuse among newly injured spinal cord patients.* Presented at the annual meeting of the Am Congress of Rehab Med, Houston, 1984.
35. MacAndrew C: Evidence for the presence of two fundamentally different, age-independent characterological types within unselected runs of male alcohol and drug abusers. *Am J Drug Alcohol Abusers* 6:207–221, 1979.
36. Adair W, Heinemann G, Donohue M, Goddard M: The relation of substance abuse and spinal cord injury onset. Presented at the annual meeting of the Am Congress of Rehab Med, Kansas City, 1985.
37. Guttmann L: Reflections on sport for the physically handicapped. *Physiotherapy* 51:252–253, 1965.
38. Buck F, Hohmann G: Personality, behavior, values, and family relations of children of fathers with spinal cord injury. *Arch Phys Med Rehabil* 62:432–438, 1981.
39. Buck F, Hohmann G: Child adjustment as related to severity of paternal disability. *Arch Phys Med Rehabil* 63:249–253, 1982.
40. Berscheid E, Walster E: Physical attractiveness. *Adv Exper Soc Psychol* 7:157–215, 1974.
41. El Ghatit A, Hanson R: Marriage and divorce after spinal cord injury. *Arch Phys Med Rehabil* 57:470–472, 1976.
42. Hopkins M: Patterns of self-destruction among the orthopedically disabled. *Rehabil Res Pract Rev* 3:5–16, 1971.
43. Bors E: Spinal cord injury. In Wohl MG (ed.): *Long Term Illness: Management of the Chronically Ill Patient.* Philadelphia, WB Saunders, 1959, pp. 469–480.
44. Seybold J: Rehabilitation and employment status report. *Paraplegic News* 29:34–36, 1976.
45. Chanin I, Brown B: Incidence of disability and characteristics of clients closed from plan with severe spinal cord injury. *Rehabil Res Rep* 34:FY1972–1973, 1975.
46. *Comprehensive Service Needs Study.* Washington, DC, Urban institute, 1975.
47. Felton J: Blocks to employment of paralytics. *Rehabil Record* 5:35–37, 1964.

Suggested Readings

Albrecht G, Higgins P: Rehabilitation success: The inter-relationships of multiple criteria. *J Health Soc Behav* 18:36–45, 1977.
Barccha R, Stewart M, Guze S: The prevalence of alcoholism among general hospital ward patients. *Am J Psychiatry* 125(5):681–684, 1968.
Bulman R, Wortman C: Attributions of blame and coping in the "real world": Severe accident victims react to their lot. *J Personality Social Psych* 35:351–363, 1977.
Braakman R, Orban IUC, Blaauw-van Dishoek M: Information in the early stages after spinal cord injury. *Paraplegia* 14:95–100, 1976.
Cole T: Sexuality in the spinal cord injured. In Green R (ed): *Human Sexuality: A Health Practioner's Text.* Baltimore, Williams & Wilkins, 1975, pp 146–170.
Dinardo QE: *Psychological adjustment to spinal cord injury.* Ph.d. Dissertation, University of Houston, 1971.
Dunn D: *Adjustment to spinal cord injury in the rehabilitation hospital setting.* Ph.D Dissertation, University of Maryland, 1969.
Fink S, Skipper J, Hallenbeck P: Physical disability and problems in marriage. *J Marriage Fam* 30:64–74, 1968.
Frisbie J, Tun C: Drinking and spinal cord injury. *J Am Paraplegia Soc* 7:71–73, 1984.
Fullerton D, Harvey R, Klein M, Howell T: Psychiatric disorders in patients with spinal cord injuries. *Arch Gen Psychiatry* 38:1369–1371, 1981.
Gans J: Depression diagnosis in a rehabilitation hospital. *Arch Phys Med Rehabil* 62:386–389, 1981.
Green B, Pratt C, Grigsby T: Self-concept among persons with long-term spinal cord injury. *Arch Phys Med Rehab* 65:751–754, 1984.
Griffith E, Timms R and Tomko N: *Sexual problems of patients with spinal injuries: An annotated bibliography.* Cincinnati, University of Cincinnati, College of Medicine, Department of Rehabilitation, 1973.
Griffith E, Treischmann R: Sexual function in women with spinal cord injury. *Arch Phys Med Rehab* 56:8–13, 1975.

Guttmann L: Sport and the disabled. In Williams JGP (ed): *Sports Medicine*. Baltimore, Williams & Wilkins, 1962, pp 367–391.

Guttmann L: Significance of sport in rehabilitation of spinal paraplegics and tetraplegics. *JAMA* 236:195–197, 1976.

Hohmann G: Considerations in management of psycho-sexual readjustment in the cord injured male. *Rehab Psychol* 19:50–58, 1972.

Khella L, Stoner E: 101 cases of spinal cord injury. *Am J Phys Med* 56:21–32, 1977.

Klas L: *A study of the relationship between depression and factors in the rehabilitation process of the hospitalized spinal cord injured patient.* Ph.D Dissertation, University of Utah, 1970.

Kleck R: Emotional arousal in interactions with stigmatized persons. *Psychol Rep* 19:1226, 1966.

Kleck R: Physical stigma and non-verbal cues emitted in face-to-face interaction. *Human Relat* 21:19–28, 1968.

Kleck R, Ono H, Hastorf A: The effects of physical deviance upon face-to-face interaction. *Human Relat* 19:425–436, 1966.

Koshland DE (ed): *Science* 229–741, August 1985.

Lawson N: Significant events in the rehabilitation process: The spinal cord patient's point of view. *Arch Phys Med Rehabil* 59:573–579, 1978.

Michael J: Rehabilitation. In Neuringer C, Michael J (eds): *Behavior Modification in Clinical Psychology*. New York: Appleton-Century-Crofts, 1970, pp 52–85.

Morgan E, Hohmann G, Davis J: Psychosocial rehabilitation in VA spinal cord injury centers. *Rehabil Psychol* 21:3–33, 1974.

Morris V, Traver W: After the battle. *Am J Nurs* 72:97–99, 1972.

Mueller A: Psychologic factors in rehabilitation of paraplegia patients. *Arch Phys Med Rehabil* 43:151–159, 1962.

Mueller A: Personality problems of spinal cord injured. *J Consult Clin Psychol* 14:189–192, 1950.

O'Connor J, Leitner L: Traumatic quadriplegia—a comprehensive review. *J Rehabil* 37:14–20, 1971.

O'Donnell J, Cooper J, Gessner J, Shehan I, Ashley J: Alcohol, drugs, and spinal cord injury. *Alcohol Health & Res World* 27–29, 1981/1982.

Pottenger M, McKernan J, Petrie L, Weissman M, Ruben H, Newberry P: The frequency and persistence of depression symptoms in the alcohol abuser. *J New Ment Dis* 166:562–570, 1978.

Rehab Brief: Bringing research into effective focus. *National Institute of Handicapped Research* vol V, no. 6, 1982.

Seymour C: Personality and paralysis: I. Comparative adjustment of paraplegics and quadriplegics. *Arch Phys Med Rehabil* 36:691–694, 1955.

Vaillant GE, Milofolay ES: Natural history of male alcoholism: IV. Paths to recovery. *Arch Gen Psychiatry* 39: 1982.

Vash C: *The psychology of disability*. New York, Springer Publishing, 1981.

Wilcox N, Stauffer E: Follow-up of 423 consecutive patients admitted to the spinal cord centre: Rancho Los Amigos Hospital, 1 January to 31 December, 1967. *Int J Paraplegia* 10:115–122, 1972.

Wittkower E, Gingras G, Mergler L, Wigdon B, Lepine A: A combined psycho-social study of spinal cord lesions. *Can Med Assoc J* 71:109–115, 1954.

Woodbury B: Adjustment to spinal cord injury: A review of the literature, 1950–1977. *Rehabil Psychol* 22:Monograph Issue, 1978.

Woodbury B, Marguette C: A model system of psychological intervention for spinal cord injury. Presented at the American Spinal Injury Association, Denver, 1983.

Wright B: *Physical Disability—A Psychosocial Approach*. New York; Harper & Row, 1983.

CHAPTER 9

Follow-up Care

HELEN CIOSCHI, R.N., M.S.N.
WILLIAM E. STAAS, Jr., M.D.

Providing follow-up care for the person with spinal cord injury (SCI) and the family unit is and should be a continuous, lifelong process. Once discharged, the person is confronted with the realities of a SCI, its effect on every body process, and its impact on his or her daily life and the life of the family. The individual may have actively participated in hospital passes to experience the disability outside the protective hospital environment. However, once at home, the novelty of a weekend pass, numerous visitors, and multiple environmental distractions decreases. Upon discharge, the individual must settle into a new routine and an altered life-style that reflects the multifaceted aspects of the disability. Through coordinated acute and rehabilitation SCI care, the extensive needs of the individual and the family unit are recognized and addressed in preparation for discharge.

Discharge planning that begins in the acute phase of care and extends throughout rehabilitation should focus on encouraging and providing for the educational and adjustment needs of the individual and family. These educational components include managing medical and functional aspects of the disability; becoming expert in performing, delivering, and directing care; recognizing the need to seek medical help; becoming knowledgeable in all aspects of equipment need and use; and identifying, seeking support, and dealing with stressors of the disability.

Overview of Follow-Up Care

Follow-up care should provide the individual with a resource when a question arises, an emergency situation develops, or there is a shared fear or concern. It should provide for formal comprehensive evaluations after discharge from the hospital. In addition, it may permit informal nursing assessments, equipment evaluations, telephone problem solving and triaging, and other unscheduled contacts initiated by the individual or family when a concern or issue arises. Patient or family needs reflect the possible and actual problems or complications of a disability, as well as the alterations accompanying a life-style change for any individual. Their needs also reinforce to the health care provider the importance of health maintenance in the biopsychosocial aspect of their daily lives.

One of the primary goals of a follow-up program should be to provide services, options, and guidelines that will assist the individual and family in achieving and maintaining a high level of health and independence. Throughout the hospitalization and rehabilitation process, preventive health maintenance and early intervention education are essential to foster optimal health throughout the individual's lifetime. Reinforcing these survival components in follow-up will assist the individual and family in attaining wellness, promoting readjustment to health, and optimizing reintegration into the community.

Follow-up care should provide a link between a comprehensive care center and the community. It should facilitate access to health care clinicians, including therapists, medical consultants, primary care providers, physiatrists, social workers, psychologists, and nurses. It is the link between the individual and community resources, including crisis intervention centers, substance abuse programs, community nursing agencies, insurance providers, recreational and vocational programs, and centers for independent living. The common goal shared by the follow-up service system and these providers is to facilitate independence and optimal health for the individual.

Discharge Preparation

Active participation in follow-up care should begin with a predischarge meeting with the patient and family and the follow-up nurse clinician. At this time, the purpose, functions, and goals of the planned follow-up program should be discussed in detail. The resources that can be provided should be reviewed fully. Explaining the role of the follow-up system as one that will assist with the ongoing and lifetime management of the disability may help alleviate some fears and concerns regarding life after hospitalization.

Areas of concern that are addressed before discharge should include the discharge plan established with the patient by the entire rehabilitation team, including the individual's disposition; the primary caregivers and their knowledge base regarding SCI and management; an accessible family practitioner, software supplier, and drugstore; equipment prescribed and to be received; the amount of professional and attendant care required; other support issues existing for the individual and family unit; the individual's need and access to community resources, including recreational and social outlets; and transportation issues, including "how to" steps for arranging and solving transportation problems.

Before discharge, it is important to include the insurance specialist in the spinal cord patient's management and discharge plan. Defining and justifying the need for home modifications, special or modified equipment, software, continuous health care, skilled or attendant care, and comprehensive follow-up management will firmly establish for the insurance provider the discharge and follow-up plan that will assist in management of patient needs in follow-up.

Providing education and training to the community health and nursing agency about the home care of the person with SCI is also essential to a successful discharge and follow-up plan. The nurse/attendants/therapists assisting the individual must be well versed in all aspects of SCI management and problem solving. They also need to recognize and utilize the follow-up system of care as a direct resource available to them for consultation and education.

A person with a SCI who is without family members or a "solid" disposition may need to be placed in an extended care facility or, if possible, an independent living situation. The rehabilitation and follow-up team need to work closely with these facilities to assist with initial adjustment and ongoing follow-up care, as well as staff education, before the patient is discharged. The follow-up system can help develop an environment that will foster the greatest level of independence while encouraging the individual to be as independent or directive in his or her care as possible.

Obviously, spinal cord follow-up care should involve more than a clinic visit. It should be a comprehensive approach to providing lifetime care that facilitates life in the community by coordinating, educating, and systematizing multiple resources with a common goal—maximizing and improving the life of the individual with spinal cord injury and of his or her family.

A System Approach to Follow-Up

FORMAL CLINIC VISITS

Beginning with the initial follow-up clinic visit, the person with SCI should have repeated neurologic and functional evaluations. These parameters are necessary in order to establish an accurate diagnosis and prognosis. The diagnosis relates primarily to neurologic level of injury and completeness or incompleteness of injury. Prognosis is dependent upon diagnosis and includes medical, functional, psychosocial, vocational, and neurologic findings.

The patient assessments are of importance not only during the acute phase of management but also during follow-up because follow-up means a lifetime commitment to the patient by the follow-up system. Improvement or regression can only be determined by repetitive, accurate examinations with documentation. The major types of assessments are motor examinations, sensory evaluation, and reflex examination.

The motor examination is more reliable and objective than is the sensory examination. It should include all major muscle groups from proximal to distal in the upper and lower extremities, as well as the thorax and abdomen.

The sensory examination is subjective and is influenced by patient cooperation. The modalities tested should include pin, light touch, and joint position sense. The dermatomes from C2 to S5 should be included. To maximize the reliability of examinations, the patient's eyes should be covered.

Tendon reflexes, including the brachioradialis, biceps, triceps, knee, and ankle, should be tested and recorded. Plantar response should be tested and notation made indicating upgoing toe, downgoing toe, or no response. The bulbocavernosus (S2–S4) and anocutaneous (S5) reflexes should also be tested. They are of critical importance in assessing neurologic status and aiding in functional prognosis.

Assessing the presence or absence of spasticity and clonus completes the basic neurologic examination. The information obtained permits the clinician to determine accurately the level of lesion and completeness or incompleteness of the lesion. Repeat examinations are important in order to recognize change in the neurologic status.

It is recommended that the patient be evaluated after discharge in a formal clinic visit at 1, 3, 6, and 12 months and yearly thereafter.

If a patient is referred to a follow-up system from another facility, medical records should be obtained and a thorough review of the records and patient assessment carried out. On initial examination, a diagnosis and functional prognosis should be determined. Understanding the functional significance of the level of spinal injury assists in determining the expected outcome and needs. Spinal stability or instability must be determined, as well as basic medical needs, functional retraining needs, and necessary adaptive equipment.

Throughout the follow-up process, the rehabilitation team must offer ongoing support for basic medical needs, including prescriptions for medications, as well as software and durable equipment. In addition, environmental modifications may require periodic revisions, depending upon patient need.

Patient and family teaching and coordinating activities with community resources, including the family physician, are of utmost importance. The family physician must be part of the team and should be in communication with key members of the rehabilitation team, including the managing physiatrist and nurse and therapists.

At each visit to the follow-up system, the patient should be evaluated by the physiatrist, the nurse, and a social worker. Depending upon need, the patient may also be evaluated by a physical or occupational therapist, rehabilitation psychologist, rehabilitation counselor, vocational evaluator and counselor, or recreational therapist.

Laboratory studies should be performed on a regular basis during the follow-up phase, based upon patient need. Particular emphasis should be placed on the genitourinary system and other major organ systems primarily susceptible to severe complications.

In summary, the formal clinic follow-up visit should be utilized for multidisciplinary patient problem identification. If necessary, regular informal clinic appointments or referrals to appropriate consultants may be recomended for problem management.

INFORMAL FOLLOW-UP VISITS

Informal follow-up visits may be necessary for the treatment of complications that were identified during the formal clinic visits. At these visits, the nurse clinician and physiatrist should manage the patient's bowel, bladder, and skin problems; do a thorough assessment of other presenting problems; and provide any additional education that the patient or family may need.

The nurse clinician should be the primary contact person in the follow-up system so that duplication of care is reduced and coordination of care among the entire follow-up team and community is enhanced. Ongoing consultation with physicians regarding specific patient care management issues allows the individual's treatment plan to be modified when necessary. Collaboration with other team members, including the social worker, psychologists, physical therapist, and occupational therapist, may be necessary to address specific therapeutic issues.

ONE SYSTEM'S EXPERIENCE

The table summarizes the experience of one regional SCI center's follow-up system during calendar year 1984. Each patient was contacted by telephone and mail to establish and confirm the schedule of appointments. If an appointment was missed, the patient was contacted, and every effort was made to prevent another absence. Patients who moved to another region were routinely referred to another SCI center for follow-up care.

The major medical/nursing and psychosocial problems described in the table demonstrate the need to help the person with SCI injury and family confront and manage the health and social realities of the disability. Providing a basic understanding of strategies to maintain health and avoid these biopsychosocial problems further reduces or prevents the need for costly readmission to the hospital and loss of time from school, work, or the family unit.

The success of the follow-up system is demonstrated in its utilization by the person with SCI, the family, and community agencies as validated in the overall statistics. A total of 664 individuals were followed by the system, and 577 of these individuals arrived for a formal clinic visit when scheduled. Some of the primary reasons for cancellations include transportation, illness, or "other" family problems. During the year, 2000 telephone contacts were made to the nurse

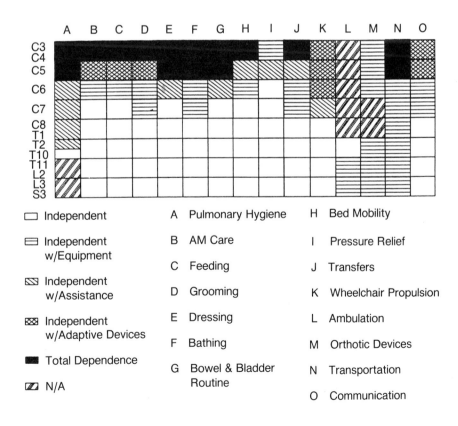

	Independent	A	Pulmonary Hygiene	H	Bed Mobility
	Independent w/Equipment	B	AM Care	I	Pressure Relief
		C	Feeding	J	Transfers
	Independent w/Assistance	D	Grooming	K	Wheelchair Propulsion
	Independent w/Adaptive Devices	E	Dressing	L	Ambulation
		F	Bathing	M	Orthotic Devices
	Total Dependence	G	Bowel & Bladder Routine	N	Transportation
	N/A			O	Communication

clinicians regarding clarification/problem solving with various aspects of care, such as bowel, bladder, and skin programs; early intervention for medical problems; and triaging acute medical problems to the system's emergency room or to a nearby hospital. The follow-up nurses also made contacts with the primary care physician, nurses/attendants, therapist, insurance specialist, suppliers, and pharmacies.

Coordinating care among all members of the spinal cord injured person's community team facilitated optimal care delivery and decreased the actual and potential complications in the individual's long-term care management.

Complications in Follow-up

GENITOURINARY

Urinary tract infections are often seen in the spinal cord injured person during the follow-up phase of care. Many males return home either voiding spontaneously or on infrequent intermittent catheterizations, i.e., every 8–12 hr or less. However, an increased incidence of infection may be seen with individuals using external collecting devices and indwelling catheters.

All individuals with indwelling catheters are subject to bacteriuria within 48 hr of insertion. The decision to treat an individual is based on a positive culture with accompanying symptomatology. Other factors influencing bladder infection development include the patient's hygiene, use of clean versus sterile technique, adequate hydration, frequency of catheter change and management, recurrent history of bladder infections, and evidence of reflux and other genitourinary dysfunctions. Individuals discharged on an intermittent catheterization program require close outpatient management through the follow-up system.

Other bladder-related problems requiring follow-up management include maintaining an external collecting device, development of an optimal bladder program for the disabled woman, episodes of dysreflexia with voiding that may indicate vesicoureteral reflux, stones, and outlet obstruction. Bladder management problems may require referral to a urologist for further investigation and management.

An annual genitourinary work-up is essential for continuous monitoring of the spinal cord injured person's genitourinary health status. Annual renal scans or intravenous pyelograms, urine cultures, and 24-hr urine for creatinine clearance provide a baseline for monitoring, treating, and, it is hoped, preventing serious urinary tract disease.

MUSCULOSKELETAL

Spasticity remains a major problem for the spinal cord injured person during the follow-up years. Spasticity may assist the person with activities of daily living (ADL), or it may be severe enough to interrupt daily functioning. The individual who presents with severe spasticity may experience sleep disturbances; interference with grooming, dressing, positioning, and transfers; skin breakdown; and contractures.

The etiology of the spasticity needs to be determined because spasticity increases in the presence of an infection, skin breakdown, or other medical problems. Treatment for the spasticity may be limited to instructing the individual to increase the range of motion (ROM) activities; altering medication regimens; and, as a last resort, surgical intervention, including rhizotomies and dorsal column stimulators.

Assessment of the individual's response to the therapeutic intervention is essential. Spasticity should be reduced to a level that will eliminate problems with ADL but not prevent the completion of them.

Contractures resulting from lack of daily ROM exercise or severe spasticity further complicate the daily health and activity of the person. Contractures interfere with ADL, positioning, and skin integrity. Prevention of contractures through proper positioning and following through on the prescribed exercise program must be a part of the individual's daily routine. All individuals involved in delivering care to the person with SCI must view these activities as an integral part of the daily routine.

Joint and muscle pain is observed in the SCI population and may be a result of improper positioning, improper wheelchair fit, performance of other daily activities, and/or the degenerative diseases of aging. Evaluating the individual's positioning, use of lap boards, chair propulsion, and daily activities provides information needed to intervene for this problem. The use of cold or heat, analgesics, and equipment adjustments if necessary may help alleviate or reduce the incidence of these problems.

Heterotopic ossification is occasionally seen in the follow-up population. Commonly described etiologic factors include trauma, edema, and vascular changes. Early signs and symptoms may include a decrease in range of motion, local swelling, and warmth. The clinician suspecting heterotopic ossification should also consider the possibility of a deep vein thrombophlebitis because the presenting symptomatology is often similar. Heterotopic ossification can greatly reduce the independence of the person as a result of restricted ROM that interferes with ADL, including transfers, seating, sitting, and dressing. Aggressive passive ROM helps reduce the contractures and deformities. Managing this problem may require initiating and/or adjusting the medication (diphosphonates), outpatient physical therapy, and reinforcing the importance of ROM activities to the individual and care providers.

PRESSURE SORES

Skin problems are a major follow-up problem that affects not only the medical health status of the individual but also his or her entire social and psychological health. Pressure sores interfere with the individual's life-style, often cause the loss of work or school days, and may require repeated and lengthy hospitalization. Grade I or II pressure sores can be healed by early treatment and conservative measures. Grades III and IV sores often require surgical intervention.

Spinal cord injured individuals who are educated about skin management, prevention of skin breakdown, and the importance of early intervention should have the knowledge base to act and respond promptly to suspicious areas. Often in follow-up care, psychosocial factors greatly influence the self-care initiated in response to a developing or present sore. Being unable to get off the area completely is a concern for the individual who lives alone or who feels that a loss of work or school days is too great a sacrifice, even if it provides for more rapid wound healing and prevents progression of the sore.

Anderson and Andberg demonstrated the relationship between pressure sores and psychosocial factors. Individuals who scored high in satisfaction with social activities and self-esteem had a decreased incidence of pressure sores. A higher incidence of sores was also seen in paraplegics, rather than quadriplegics. Quadriplegics are most likely to have another individual assuming responsibility for their daily care, including skin management, whereas paraplegics who are expected to be independent with self-care may not identify maintaining skin integrity as an ongoing major priority in their day-to-day activities.

Ongoing education remains an important factor in maintaining healthy skin. Being aware of prevention measures and actually incorporating them into their daily routine are essential components of daily care for spinal cord injured persons.

Some SCI centers offer pressure sore readmission programs that provide behavioral and educational components at the same time as the delivery of the necessary medical/surgical and rehabilitative care for persons who cannot be optimally managed on an outpatient basis. During the hospital stay, the individual participates in a comprehensive rehabilitation program while learning to modify his or her response to factors in the environment that contributed to the pressure sore development. Classes on managing everyday life concerns, such as stress, assertiveness training, effects of substance abuse, and how to seek help, may also be provided. The overall goal is to effect a behavioral and attitudinal change toward maintaining optimal health and skin integrity that will prevent the recurrence of pressure sores.

GASTROINTESTINAL

Difficulties with bowel routines in the follow-up population may be related to alterations in diet, activity level, method and changes of bowel routine, and problems with attendant care. Once home, the person with SCI may have to rearrange his or her routine, eating, and activity habits to fit into the family life, attendant care, work, or school schedule. Assistance with modifying the program based on these new needs is provided through the follow-up system.

During the follow-up period, the individual may be gradually weaned from bowel medications until digital stimulation and increasing abdominal pressure and abdominal massage produce effective results. The individual should be knowledgeable in all aspects of the routine, including problem-solving activities. These problem situations should be discussed with the patient at clinic visits to ensure that appropriate interventions can be initiated when necessary.

Nutritional concerns or changes in eating habits are a problem not only for the adolescent but also for the elderly patient. Anorexia, a common problem in adolescence, may be noted during the follow-up phase. Possible causes include medication side effects, depression, and lack of interest in eating due to social reasons. Assessing eating habits, meal preparation, and quality and quantity of food intake is essential in monitoring the nutritional status of the spinal cord injured person. Body weights, complete blood count, serum protein, and overall assessment of the individual's health provide a baseline for nutritional assessment on an ongoing basis.

Obesity also presents multiple problems for the individual. Excess weight gain impairs the individual's ability to perform ADL, makes transfers difficult, may require a change in equipment to avoid pressure sores and positioning problems, and may significantly reduce the activity level of the person. Depression over the weight gain may also compound the existing depression and impede adaptation to the losses resulting from the injury. The individual's family may have substituted food for activity and recreational diversion, which further increases the weight and accompanying psychosocial problem. Recreational diversion; finding new substitutes for food or providing low-calorie, high fiber/bulk foods; and reducing snacking between meals are conservative interventions.

Nutritional and psychological counseling may also be indicated for the person with an eating disorder. Referral to a specialized eating disorder program and working collaboratively with that program may help the individual deal with and solve this problem.

Spinal cord injured persons must also realize that they are not immune to heart disease or hypertension and that they should modify their diet accordingly if early signs of these conditions arise.

Gastrointestinal disturbances include hiatal hernia, stress ulcers, gallbladder disease, and liver dysfunction. Perhaps as the population ages, an increase in the incidence of gastrointestinal disorders may be observed. Assessing for these problems, as well as referral to an internist or gastroenterologist, may be required.

MEDICATION MANAGEMENT

The person with SCI often requires ongoing management of the medication regimens, including close regulation of antispasticity, pain, bladder, or bowel medications. The physician and clinician's role in medication management should be to evaluate the effectiveness of the regimen and to modify it as necessary. It is essential that the person with SCI understand the purpose, action, and side effects of the drug regimen and report any suspected or actual adverse drug reactions promptly. Working collaboratively with the family physician enables close supervision of the drug regimen and avoids overmedication.

NEUROSENSORY

In this population, there is a high incidence of chronic pain, especially in those individuals with lumbosacral and cauda equina lesions. The pain is usually reported as chronic numbness and tingling in areas of the body that are insensate on neurologic examinations.

Pain needs to be thoroughly evaluated to determine its origin and nature and to ensure an appropriate therapeutic regimen. Individuals experiencing pain may receive moderate relief from tricyclic antidepressants given alone or in combination with pheonothiazines. Other pain management modalities include counseling, TENS units, relaxation techniques, and guided imagery that may be effective alone or used in conjunction with a medication regimen.

Neurosensory pain in those individuals with spared sensation may also be a manifestation of a chronic disease, especially in the elderly client who may be susceptible to other neuropathies. This reinforces the need to consider all possible spinal cord and nonspinal cord pathologies that may influence the development of neurosensory pain.

CARDIOVASCULAR

Cardiovascular complications, including alterations in blood pressure regulation and dependent edema, are common problems in the follow-up years. Educating the individual about preventive measures, including gradual positioning change, use of an abdominal binder and elastic stockings, and maintaining adequate salt and fluid intake helps regulate blood pressure.

Edema usually results from the lower extremities (and upper extremities in the person with quadriplegia) being in a dependent position. Edema that is absent upon awakening, but progresses throughout the day is dependent in origin. The individual should be instructed to elevate the lower extremities, perform passive ROM exercises, and use elastic stockings; if edema persists, the use of elevating legrests on the wheelchair may be indicated.

A more serious and life-threatening problem, deep vein thrombophlebitis (DVT), is seen infrequently during the follow-up years, but can occur even 2–3 years or more after the initial trauma. Signs and symptoms of DVT must be a part of the individual's knowledge base upon discharge. The importance of seeking prompt medical attention if these signs and symptoms are experienced should be emphasized. Patients with a previous history of phlebitis and Greenfield filter insertion also need prompt evaluation if signs and symptoms occur because filters can become displaced. The patient suspected of having a phlebitis should be instructed to stop ROM activities, maintain bedrest, and seek emergency care for diagnostic evaluation. Readmission for anticoagulation therapy is indicated.

RESPIRATORY

Respiratory problems, including upper and lower respiratory tract infections, are common occurrences in persons with quadriplegia and high-level paraplegia. Emphasis on maintaining good pulmonary hygiene by performing deep breathing and assistive coughing techniques is essential. The use of triflow and adequate hydration and the need to avoid individuals with infections should also be reinforced.

Recognition of the early signs of respiratory tract infection and prompt intervention should be strongly encouraged. The administration of pneumovax and an annual flu vaccine may further reduce the incidence of pulmonary infections in this population.

Pulmonary embolus, although rare, can occur any time following injury, but especially postoperatively or after prolonged periods of immobilization/bedrest during the follow-up years. Signs and symptoms may be altered in this population. Any evidence of tachypnea, chest pain, or abrupt onset of shoulder pain should be thoroughly evaluated for possible embolus.

SEXUAL/REPRODUCTIVE

Sexual and reproductive issues are common concerns of the person with a SCI during the follow-up years. These issues take on more importance when the individual returns home or to an environment that facilitates relationship building. Concerns include fertility, performance issues, and sexual adjustment to the various components of the disability, i.e., bowel/bladder routines.

Individual and joint counseling should be provided by the nurse clinician, physician, and/or social worker with consultations to appropriate specialists when necessary. Females with SCI should be provided adequate and appropriate contraceptive information and counseling. Providing instruction on breast and testicular examinations, emphasizing the need for annual pelvic exams, and providing information on sexually transmitted diseases are important roles in follow-up health maintenance.

FUNCTIONAL

Mobility issues for the person with SCI in follow-up are specifically related to wheelchair usage and ambulation training. The patient may require further evaluation for equipment or other mobility issues. Equipment needs are evaluated during a formal equipment clinic by a physical therapist spinal cord specialist, along with the nurse clinician and physician. The person with quadriplegia may be evaluated for the use of a motorized wheelchair to enhance mobility at school or work. Equipment that could improve the functional ability of individuals new to the follow-up system may have never been considered in the past, or possibly a new funding source may have been identified, permitting the individual to obtain or rent the necessary items. Throughout the follow-up years, equipment will require repair, and evaluation for new equipment may be necessary based on a change in the person's functional status.

PSYCHOSOCIAL/VOCATIONAL PROBLEMS

Addressing the psychosocial realities and complexities of adaptation to the disability requires ongoing comprehensive support, utilization of peer/support groups, and psychological counseling. Difficulties with adjusting and adapting to the disability are manifested and identified in the individual, as well as the family unit, and both require ongoing support and intervention.

Identifying and utilizing the spinal cord center and community resources are of paramount importance in enabling the individual to re-establish some degree of control and adaptation. Assisting the patient and family in developing appropriate coping and problem-solving skills may also help reduce the incidence of maladaptive behavior, such as substance abuse, which further complicates the biopsychosocial health of the individual.

Psychological counseling should be provided, and if necessary, appropriate referrals to psychiatrists and community centers should be made. Other problems of major concern for this population include financial problems that are increased by the disability, transportation, accessible housing, and inadequate recreational and social outlets that impede adaptation and adjustment.

Abuse of drugs and alcohol further impairs the biopsychosocial health of the person with SCI and the family. The individual may use this pharmacologic escape to deal with the long-term emotional issues of the disability. Habitual drug use may also further impair the total well-being of the individual, causing medical and other disability problems, such as skin problems, which are avoidable. The need to identify individuals with a preinjury history of substance abuse and to work with them in managing this problem is essential in preventing recurrence after discharge from the hospital. Utilization of community resources, including detoxification and drug rehabilitation programs and individual/family support groups, is critical to treating and addressing this serious problem.

Readmission to the Hospital

Urinary tract infections and pressure sore problems are the major causes for readmission to the hospital for persons with SCI. A small percentage of individuals require multiple readmissions to the hospital within a calendar year, whereas the majority do not require any readmissions to the hospital. Most readmissions are to the SCI center's acute or rehabilitation hospitals. Readmission to outside hospitals requires contact from the follow-up system to ensure maintenance of specific programs for the individual, i.e., respiratory, bowel, bladder, and skin care. Hospital readmissions may increase in the future as the SCI population ages and specific age-related illnesses and problems become more evident.

Health Maintenance Issues

Obviously, health maintenance issues are an integral part of the care for the person with SCI from the onset of injury and throughout his or her lifetime. Focusing only on the disability-related issues and needs may obscure the need for a total health plan for the person with SCI. Appropriate immunizations, vaccines, and screening measures for malignancy and cardiovascular disease should be an integral component of spinal cord follow-up care.

If a primary care provider is not available or accessible to the individual, his or her health maintenance needs may need to be assumed by the follow-up system with appropriate referral to general/family medicine. As health care providers, it is important to remember that the person with SCI is just as susceptible to age- and environment-related problems and should actively participate and receive health prevention/maintenance activities.

Special Subgroups in the SCI Population

Spinal cord injured females, although only 20% of the SCI population, have special needs and health issues related to the disability and their general well-being that need closer attention and research. Further exploration of sexuality and sexual function from the menstrual through postmenopausal years is essential. Community support services providing for the needs of the disabled woman should be developed and utilized. Adaptations in providing for their health care needs, such as enlarging gynecologic examination rooms, accessibility of high-low tables, providing assistive devices for hygiene and contraceptive needs, modifying techniques for self-breast examinations, and providing an atmosphere of wellness for the disabled woman, are essential.

Spinal cord injuries commonly occur in the elderly as a result of falls. When managing the elderly person with SCI, the health care provider needs to consider age-related and disability-related problems. Prevention and health maintenance issues are important. Ongoing management of chronic disease processes, along with the alterations resulting from the SCI, requires a coordinated effort among the entire hospital and community health care team. Responding to the needs of this special population requires a multidisciplinary approach with support from agencies for the aging. Providing support to the spouse or significant other providing care for this individual is also important, because many of these individuals may be physically unable to care for the individual or may become unable to assist with home care. If nursing home placement is necessary, working collaboratively with the agency to provide for the needs of this individual as a person with SCI helps provide a higher quality of care that addresses all actual or potential needs and problems.

Comprehensive spinal cord management initiated from the onset of injury and throughout lifetime follow-up care has increased the longevity of the person with SCI. However, these extended lifetimes demand more than efforts to reduce readmissions and lengths-of-stays. Through the collaborative efforts of the patient and family with other system and community health providers, the multiple needs and concerns of individuals with a SCI can be confronted and managed. Increasing the life span of the spinal cord injured person may achieve statistical significance. However, attempting to improve the quality of life along with the increase in survival years through comprehensive follow-up management remains an ongoing challenge and responsibility for the entire health care team.

Suggested Readings

Anderson TP, Andberg MM: Psychosocial factors associated with pressure sores. *Arch Phys Med Rehab* 60:341, 1979.

Ruskin A: *Current Therapy in Physiatry.* Philadelphia, WB Saunders, 1984, pp 379–457.

Williams, TF: *Rehabilitation in the Aging.* New York, Raven Press, 1984.

CHAPTER 10

Spinal Cord Regeneration

SCOTT A. MACKLER, M.D., Ph.D.
MICHAEL E. SELZER, M.D., Ph.D.

The devastating loss of motor and sensory functions that occurs following spinal cord injury (SCI) in humans was recognized more than 4000 years ago, as described in the Edwin Smith Surgical Papyrus. However, interest in experiments studying the responses of the central nervous system (CNS) to injury and the possibility of subsequent regeneration did not, in large part, develop until the late 19th century. During the past 100 years many laboratories have examined the question of whether or not functional regeneration occurs in the vertebrate CNS. This chapter reviews the major results and conclusions developed during this time period.

Early in this century Ramon y Cajal, a major figure in modern neurobiology, demonstrated that transected nerve fibers in the spinal cords of young mammals first died back and then regenerated for short distances, but did not grow past the original lesion site. This concept of abortive regeneration has been consistently confirmed. Improvements in various techniques—notably those of intracellular dye markers, electrophysiologic recordings, and cell culture—have led to an explosion in information concerning the neurosciences, including the field of CNS regeneration. This has raised the hopes that a treatment program designed to restore lost function in the spinal cord injured patient can someday be realized.

Questions raised by regeneration studies are broad in nature, but the more academic issues are overshadowed by the existence of an expanding population of persons with SCI, presently estimated at over 200,000 worldwide.

The pressure from a society caring for such a large number of permanently disabled citizens has revitalized the search for a successful treatment of lost function. Theoretically, the most direct approach would be to aid the regeneration of transected nerve fibers through and/or around the scar site.

Ethical and technical problems prevent systematic approaches in experiments designed to enhance regeneration in the spinal cord of humans. This lack of properly designed prospective clinical studies has resulted in the use of numerous nonhuman mammalian models. Unfortunately, many reports in the past have generated more heat than light in demonstrating the existence of functional regeneration. A fair conclusion at the present time is that no clear evidence exists in any mammal for the permanent recovery of lost behavior following a complete spinal cord transection. In direct contrast to this fact are the many examples of behavioral recovery in nonmammalian vertebrates after spinal transection. A detailed understanding of the factors involved in the dramatic return of function in these animals, coupled with efforts to enhance regeneration in mammals, may someday lead to a successful treatment program for the person with SCI.

Mechanisms of Functional Recovery

Functional regeneration can be defined as the return of any behavior, which was eliminated by previous injury, that is the result of nerve fiber regeneration. The causal relationship between axonal regeneration and behavioral recovery must be unequivocal and must meet specific criteria that have been formulated.

The criteria for functional spinal cord regeneration are (1) the lesion must be complete, (2) fibers must grow past the scar, (3) the new fibers must contact neurons on the opposite side of the scar, (4) activation of the regenerated fiber must elicit a response in neurons on the opposite side of the scar, and (5) these newly formed connections must underlie the behavioral recovery.

At least four ways exist in which neurons can regenerate following a complete transection (Fig. 10.1). The original pattern is depicted in Figure 10.1A. Fusion of the proximal segment of a damaged axon to its surviving distal stump ensures precise matching of pre- and post-synaptic neurons; it sometimes occurs in invertebrates (Fig. 10.1B). It has never been observed in vertebrates, where the distal segment is always eliminated (Wallerian degeneration). The proximal segment may itself send fibers that grow far enough to contact their original postsynaptic targets (Fig. 10.1C). This long distance, point-to-point regeneration would require growth in the mammalian CNS on the order of centimeters. However, shorter distances of growth—that is, millimeters—by a regenerating fiber could enable it to emerge just beyond the lesion site to form novel connections that result in behavioral recovery (Fig. 10.1D). Finally, previously undamaged neurons can send out new fibers and compensate for lost connections by strengthening or supplementing remaining ones (Fig. 10.1E). This phenomenon, known as collateral sprouting, occurs in the mammalian CNS and may play a significant role in return of function after an incomplete transection.

Nervous system damage early in an organism's development usually does not result in as extensive a neurologic deficit as does injury to an adult CNS. This is partly because neurons may still possess the ability to divide and send out neurites into a relatively primitive environment. However, SCI in humans almost always occurs in a fully differentiated nervous system consisting of a stable number of post-mitotic cells. For this reason, it is practical to emphasize only those experiments that employ a spinal cord with a stable neuronal structure.

Regeneration in Nonmammalian Vertebrates

Functional regeneration occurs more vigorously not only in animals that are younger but also in those that appeared earlier during evolution. Return of motor and sensory behavior has been commonly observed in cyclostomes, teleost fish, and certain amphibians. Higher vertebrates are probably not capable of functional regeneration in the spinal cord. Studies in reptiles have mostly relied upon whole tail amputation. This results in ependymal proliferation and the formation of new neurons, which is not a true example of axonal regeneration. Rare reports of birds recovering the ability to walk after spinal cord

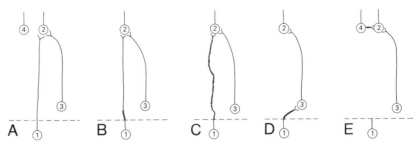

Figure 10.1. Mechanisms of functional recovery. Regenerated segments are depicted as darker uneven lines. *A*, Original pattern. *B*, Fusion of proximal and distal segments. *C*, Long distance regeneration. *D*, Short distance regeneration. *E*, collateral sprouting.

transection have been characterized by inaccurate and poorly controlled methods.

The large larval sea lamprey (up to 5 years old) has a CNS nearly identical to its adult counterpart. This cyclostome (a jawless fish) regains the ability to swim and respond to sensory stimuli 6–8 weeks after a complete spinal cord transection. Axons regenerate for short distances beyond the scar and stop growing. Therefore, they cannot contact most of the distal and original postysynaptic targets. Nevertheless, the recovered behaviors are almost indistinguishable from those of an unoperated larva. The regenerated fibers form functioning monosynaptic contacts with neurons on the opposite side of the lesion. Not surprisingly, this primitive vertebrate is the first experimental preparation to fulfill all of the criteria established for functional spinal cord regeneration.

The return of swimming in bony fish may rely upon a mechanism other than the short distances of growth observed in the larval sea lamprey. Regeneration of spinal axons proceeds for long distances—centimeters versus the limited growth of millimeters observed in the lamprey—past the healed scar and may represent point-to-point regeneration. Among amphibians, both larval and adult forms of the more primitive urodoeles (salamanders) demonstrate behavioral recovery after spinal transection. However, only the larvae of the more advanced anurans (frogs and toads) are equal in an ability to recover from spinal cord injury. It is not yet clear how far the regenerating axons in either amphibian order grow past the scar.

Any discussion of axonal regeneration should include a brief description of the classical studies of Sperry and others in optic nerve regeneration. Bony fish, urodoeles, and anurans all recover visual function after complete optic nerve section. The regenerating axons from the retinal ganglion cells grow all the way to their original target tissue and appear to innervate appropriate postsynaptic cells selectively from a multitude of others. This is the most dramatic example of true point-to-point regeneration in the vertebrate phylum. In comparison to regenerating spinal axons, however, the optic nerve fibers grow through an environment that is simpler and more conducive to regeneration.

Studies in Mammals following Complete Spinal Transection

Ramon y Cajal's detailed description of abortive regeneration in dogs and cats helped explain the lack of functional recovery that had been uniformly observed in human patients. More importantly, those experiments demonstrated that central neurons could send out newly formed fibers for short distances and that the absence of functional regeneration was simply not intrinsic to the damaged cell. Perhaps the most striking example of the role played by extrinsic factors in the success or failure of regeneration is that of the dorsal root ganglion cell (Fig. 10.2). Interruption of the peripheral process is followed by axonal regeneration over long distances, similar to findings in other peripheral nerve fibers. However, cutting the central process results in regrowth up to, but not beyond, the peripheral nervous system-CNS boundary. Clearly, failure of regeneration of the axon of the dorsal root ganglion neuron into the CNS is not a consequence of the cell's inability to regenerate, but rather other extrinsic factors are involved.

Work in the four decades following Ramon y Cajal's monograph in large part reaffirmed the finding of abortive regeneration in dogs, cats, rodents, and monkeys. The few reports of return of motor function after SCI involved the use of fetal or very young mammals that may have received incomplete transections. As previously mentioned, these experiments may not bear much relevance to the present population of spinal cord injured patients. In addition, other investigators have not been able to repeat these experiments successfully.

Some examples of unaided axonal regeneration do exist in selected areas of the mammalian CNS. These include neurosecretory fibers of the posterior pituitary gland, olfactory neurons in the nasal epithelium, and central monoaminergic fibers. Some explanations have been proposed for these special exceptions. The neurosecretory axons grow in an unusual environment because of differences in the glial cells

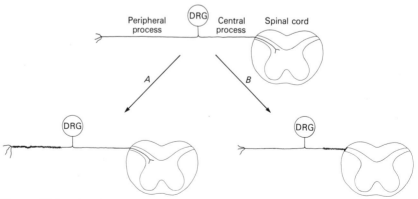

Figure 10.2. A, Cutting the peripheral process of the dorsal root ganglion cell (DRG) may be followed by successful and functional regeneration. B, Cutting the central process is not followed by regeneration into the spinal cord. Growth abruptly halts at the peripheral nervous system-CNS interface.

(pituicytes) and a more permissive blood-brain barrier. The regeneration of olfactory axons involves the division and differentiation of new neurons. The damage to monoaminergic fibers in most experiments resulted from chemical treatment and not complete transection.

EXPLANATIONS FOR THE LACK OF FUNCTIONAL REGENERATION

As evidence accumulated that regeneration of spinal axons in mammals was abortive, investigators addressed the question of what factors prevented axons from growing for significant distances. It was hoped that knowledge of what was responsible for failure of regeneration could lead to methods that might enhance axonal regeneration. Ramon y Cajal hypothesized that these factors could be divided into intrinsic and extrinsic properties of the neuron, a classification still useful today (Table 10.1). These postulated mechanisms need not be mutually exclusive.

Intrinsic neuronal properties that interfere with successful regeneration have been difficult to establish. One such property could be the axotomy-induced constellation of changes in the neuron, known as the axon reaction. Although some cells die following severance of their axon and individual neurons differ in their response to axotomy, several facts argue against this reaction as the primary impediment to functional regeneration. In nonmammalian vertebrates successful regeneration seems to be a general property of all cell types studied. The peripheral process of a dorsal root ganglion cell can regenerate over long distances, but the central process of the same cell abruptly stops at the surface of the CNS (Fig. 10.2). Differentiated neurons in a mature CNS may have lost the ability to respond to appropriate cues in the environment that regulate neurite extension and axonal growth, perhaps due to an abnormality in the components of the cell membrane. But again, the evidence does not support intrinsic failure as the major reason for incomplete regeneration.

The physical and chemical influences of the external environment most likely are more important than intrinsic properties in determining whether functional regeneration can occur. Because regenerating fibers did not grow beyond the scar tissue, many researchers felt that

Table 10.1
Reasons for the Absence of Functional Regeneration in Mammals

Intrinsic Failure of the Damaged Neuron	Factors Extrinsic to the Neuron
Axotomy-induced death	Physical barriers
Inadequate axon reaction	Glial-collagen scar
Maturation loss of ability to respond to external cues	Compact CNS
	Improper orientation
Deficiency of certain membrane components	Glial cells
	Extracellular matrix components
	Neutrotrophic molecules
	Contact inhibition
	Autoimmune damage
	Ischemia

this site acted as a physical barrier. This may in large part be true, but evidence from lower vertebrates has shown that fibers can grow through both proliferating and mature scar tissue. Other growth-inhibiting mechanical factors that have been suggested include the relative compactness of the CNS due to a small extracellular space and the improper orientation of the growing fibers.

Peripheral nerve fibers are capable of functional regeneration. A comparison between the peripheral nervous system and CNS environments has strongly implicated two components, the glial cells and the chemical structure of the extracellular space, in the ability to regenerate. Schwann cells, the glial cells unique to peripheral nerves, are intricately involved in the ability of such nerves to regenerate. The oligodendrocyte, the homologous glial cell in the CNS, differs both morphologically and biochemically. Certain glycoproteins, notably fibronectin and laminin, are secreted by fibroblasts and Schwann cells in peripheral nerves, but are not found within the parenchyma of the CNS. These compounds are not implicated as mediators of neurite adhesion and extension during development.

Trophic substances are those that aid and support axonal growth. Nerve growth factor (NGF) is the best studied and the prototypical molecule. Improved culture techniques have demonstrated the ability of many neuronal and non-neuronal cells to produce and secrete NGF and other trophic chemicals. The interaction between the advancing tip of a growing fiber and the environment it encounters is an active process, one in which all cells involved play important roles. This factor emphasizes the potential benefits of pharmacologic intervention.

An interesting hypothesis that has been proposed to explain limitations in CNS regeneration and that stresses interaction between the regenerating axon and its environment is that of contact inhibition. This hypothesis states that neurons are limited in the number of synaptic connections they can form. In the goldfish, when spinal cord regeneration was prevented by insertion of a teflon barrier at the site of the transection, many inappropriate synapses were formed by axons in the region immediately proximal to the scar. It was proposed that these synapses prevented any further regeneration because when the barrier was removed the axons did not grow any further.

Injury to the spinal cord damages the structural integrity of the blood-brain barrier, and some investigators feel that this exposes the immune system to previously unrecognized CNS autoantigens. Subsequent immune damage interferes with significant regeneration. This hypothesis is not universally accepted.

Adequate vascular supply is essential to any repair process in the body, and many have hypothesized that the unique susceptibility of the CNS to ischemia is a critical reason for the observed lack of functional regeneration. The extent of SCI is increased by interruption of the blood flow, which may damage any underlying substrate necessary for the regenerative process. Although improving the blood flow to the spinal cord may not directly enhance regeneration, this important area of potential therapy is included in the next section.

Factors—cellular or extracellular—in the environment encountered by a regenerating axon seem to dictate whether functional regeneration will occur. Most strategies developed to enhance axonal regeneration have concentrated on these suspected factors.

Attempts to Enhance Spinal Cord Regeneration

As explained above, unaided axonal regeneration does not occur in the mammalian spinal cord. Therefore, treatment strategies have been designed to circumvent the many obstacles postulated to result in abortive regeneration. Intervention—surgical and pharmacologic manipulations—has been aimed at altering intrinsic and extrinsic factors thought to impede regeneration (Table 10.2). Although some techniques are now showing promise, many of them were first attempted earlier this century.

Differentiated neurons may require assistance in redirecting their enzymatic machinery from its usual functions to regeneration. Nerve growth factor (NGF) and thyroid hormones have been given to spinal cord injured mammals because of their well-characterized anabolic effects on the developing nervous system. Paradoxically, puromycin—a protein-synthesis inhibitor—has also been used. None of these drugs in pharmacologic doses has met with consistent success.

Gangliosides are important constituents of neuronal membranes and have been implicated in some aspect of neurite extension. Intra-

Table 10.2
Strategies to Enhance Axonal Regeneration

Strategies Directed at the Neuron	Strategies Directed at the Environment
Increase anabolic reactions	Reduce glial-collagen scar
NGF	Pyrogens
Thyroid hormones	Proteolytic enzymes
Alter the axon reaction	Corticosteroids/ACTH
Puromycin	Irradiation
Cytotoxic agents (?)	Provide appropriate milieu
Replace neurons	Peripheral nerve grafts immediate or delayed
Fetal tissue transplants	NGF/other trophic molecules
Enhance neurite growth	Extracellular matrix components
Gangliosides	Millipore filter
Electrical stimulation	Vertebral resection
	Reduce ischemia
	Naloxone
	TRH
	HBO
	DMSO
	Omental transfer
	Hypothermia
	Immunosuppressive drugs
	Corticosteroids/ACTH
	Cyclophosphamide
	Azathioprine

peritoneal injection of various ganglioside preparations, a simple procedure, has stimulated growth of fibers after damage to the mammalian hippocampus and brainstem. Similar work has not yet been performed in the spinal cord injured animal. Another attractive alternative is electrical stimulation, because endogenous electrical currents are involved in the development of axonal pathways. Moreover, exogenously applied currents affect neurite growth in vitro and have enhanced distances of axonal regeneration in the lamprey spinal cord. This type of treatment has not been studied extensively in the mammalian spinal cord.

If the axotomized neuron is incapable of regeneration, why not replace it with one that is? The exciting area of neural transplantation is now being systematically explored. Nerve cells from embryonic donor animals have been successfully grafted to most regions of the mammalian neuraxis, including the spinal cord. These implants have survived and become integrated into host neuronal circuits. Substantia nigral and intracerebral grafts have even improved motor and cognitive performance in rats with previous neurologic dysfunction. The most critical requirement is that the grafts be harvested from developing (fetal and neonatal) donor nervous systems. Although this requirement may limit somewhat its applicability in SCI treatment programs, the CNS is immunologically "privileged." This means that grafts of CNS tissue from nonhuman embryonic donors might someday be used to bridge a SCI.

The glial-collagen scar has long been recognized as a major physical barrier to axonal regeneration. Attempts to reduce its formation have included local and intrathecal enzymes, steroid therapy, irradiation to prevent glial proliferation, and bacterial pyrogens. Pyrogens were chosen following experiments investigating the neural control of temperature regulation. All of these treatments do reduce the formation of the glial-collagen scar, but only for a limited time. Any observed improvements in function disappeared at later periods. In the opinion of these authors, all other treatment modalities with the possible exception of neural transplants must eventually address the problem of a restrictive scar formed either at the site of the original injury or created by any subsequent surgical procedures.

One of the most interesting treatment strategies is that of providing the appropriate milieu for axonal regeneration. Because functional regeneration occurs in the peripheral nervous system, most investigators have utilized those cellular and noncellular components of peripheral nerves that are not found in the CNS. Peripheral nerve grafts, either free at one end or bridging two regions of the neuraxis, have demonstrated that axons of central neurons can grow for long distances (up to 5 cm) within the graft. These results have included spinal axons, which clearly demonstrates that the abortive response is not fully ascribable to an intrinsic inability of CNS axons to grow. Delayed grafting—waiting 1 week after transection—has been employed in attempts to avoid a cavitation necrosis that occurs in the first few days at the site of the lesion.

Other factors that have or may be added to make the extra-axonal environment permissive to regeneration include NGF; other trophic factors; components of the extracellular matrix, such as laminin and fibronectin; and Millipore filters. The various chemicals chosen are intended to replace necessary growth factors that the adult mammalian CNS is incapable of producing in appropriate amounts. The Millipore filter paper was originally thought to help orient axons longitudinally, but actually may provide a scaffolding onto which glial cells may proliferate.

Peripheral nerve grafts and these other techniques are now being intensely investigated. The exciting finding of enhanced regeneration in a new environment needs to be studied further, because there is still no proof for significant growth of axons into the CNS parenchyma.

Vertebral resection, designed to bring surviving ends of a transected spinal cord within proximity of each other without significant tension, may not work unless combined with other treatment modalities. One such possibility is direct reanastomosis of the spinal cord.

Alleviating any ischemic damage that complicates spinal cord trauma is an important goal and one that might be critical for subsequent regeneration. Injury-induced release of endorphins is thought to be responsible for a reduction in spinal cord blood flow. The opiate antagonist naloxone and the hypothalamic peptide, thyrotropin-releasing hormone (TRH), have been injected intravenously in rats, rabbits, and cats after incomplete spinal cord contusions. An increase in the postoperative spinal cord blood flow was accompanied by a reduction in spasticity and improvements in motor function. Hyperbaric oxygen (HBO), dimethylsulfide oxide (DMSO), local hypothermia, and transfer of an omental flap onto the spinal cord surface all also have the common goal of improving blood flow and limiting the effects of intramedullary ischemia. More work needs to be completed before it can be concluded that any of these treatments produces significantly long-term improvement in outcome.

Finally, if spinal cord damage is mediated by an autoimmune process as suggested by some investigators, then modulation of this destruction may result in subsequent regeneration. Agents used include hormones of the pituitary-adrenal axis and cytotoxic agents. These experiments have not yielded satisfactory results.

SELECTED EXAMPLES OF TREATMENT IN HUMANS

A thorough search of the literature for studies designed to examine or enhance axonal regeneration in spinal cord injured patients is noteworthy for the absence of such reports. However, many individual case reports exist in which patients have been subjected to a few treatment modalities. Early in this century immediate surgical reanastomosis of a complete transection was performed in a young woman. Although records are not complete, the recovery initially recorded by the attending surgeons seems to have been either overstated or inaccurate. In another patient, sections of intercostal nerve from the periphery were anastomosed directly into the spinal cord. Optimistic preliminary reports were not reconfirmed, due to the patient's early death from an intra-abdominal abscess. Others have tried local hypothermia, possibly due to its ease of application or lack of serious side effects. The results have been inconsistent and difficult to evaluate.

There are at least two reasons for interpreting isolated case reports with caution. First, the sample populations are small and uncontrolled for the variability of the clinical course in SCI. Second, even a small remaining segment of spinal cord connecting rostral and caudal stumps can conduct significant information, re-emphasizing the need for models utilizing complete spinal transections that result in unambiguous findings.

Animal studies that have demonstrated some functional improvement from corticosteroid therapy for acute SCI have been used as a rationale for that treatment in humans. In one of the few properly performed clinical trials in human SCI, a recent double-blind, randomized study compared the efficacy of low dose versus high dose intravenous (i.v.) steroid therapy. In direct contrast to findings from animals, this study showed no differences between either treatment regimen. In fact, high dose i.v. steroids were associated with an increased risk of wound infections and possibly an increase in early fatality. These results emphasize the hazards in extending treatment modalities from animal models to humans. The assorted potential therapies listed in the previous section should be more carefully evaluated before they can be tested on human patients.

Reports from the Soviet Union have described positive results in patients treated with pyrogens and enzymes. Some patients exhibited return of sensory and minimal voluntary motor functions. Although this might represent a true benefit from intervention, it is still prudent to investigate all potential treatment regimens carefully in well-established animal models.

Conclusions

1. The growth in the number of spinal cord injured individuals demands the formulation of treatment regimens designed not only to preserve remaining neurologic function but also to restore lost motor and sensory behaviors.

2. The major hypothetical mechanism for restoring lost function is axonal regeneration and re-establishment of severed connections.

3. The spinal axons of jawless fish, bony fish, and some amphibians are unique in their ability to regenerate unaided across a scar. This regeneration is accompanied by synaptic reconnections and a dramatic behavioral recovery. A better understanding of the factors involved may aid attempts to enhance regeneration in higher vertebrates.

4. Identification of factors that interfere with regeneration has led to proposals for corrective treatment strategies aimed at achieving functional regrowth of mammalian spinal axons.

5. Procedures that show promise in enhancing axonal regeneration include peripheral nerve bridge grafting, fetal tissue transplants,

and the addition of various molecules designed to augment the extra-axonal environment.

6. At the present time no clear evidence exists for the permanent return of lost function following complete spinal transection in any mammal, regardless of treatment.

Suggested Readings

Clemente CD: Regeneration in the vertebrate central nervous system. *Int Rev Neurobiol* 6:257–302. 1964.

Gaze RM: Regeneration of the optic nerve in Amphibia. *Int Rev Neurobiol* 2:1–40, 1960.

Jacobson M, Gaze RM: Types of visual response from single units in the optic tectum and optic nerve of the goldfish. *Q J Exp Physiol* 49:199–209, 1964.

Kao CC, Bunge RP, Reier PJ (eds): *Spinal Cord Reconstruction*. New York, Raven Press, 1982.

Mackler SA, Seizer ME: Regeneration of functional synapses between individual recognizable neurons in the lamprey spinal cord. *Science* 229:774–776, 1985.

Puchala E, Windle WF: The possibility of structural and functional restitution after spinal cord injury. A review. *Exp Neurol* 55:1–42, 1977.

Ramon y Cajal S: *Degeneration and Regeneration of the Nervous System* (R.M. May transl.). London, Oxford University Press 1928.

Selzer ME: Mechanisms of functional recovery and regeneration after spinal cord transection in larval sea lampreys. *J Physiol (London)* 277:395–408, 1978.

Selzer ME: Peripheral nerve regeneration. In Sumner AJ (Ed): *The Physiology of Peripheral Nerve Disease*. Philadelphia, WB Saunders, 1981.

Sperry RW: Optic nerve regeneration with return to vision in anurans. *J Neurophysiol* 7:57–69, 1944.

Sperry RW: Chemoaffinity in the orderly growth of nerve fiber patterns and connections. *PNAS (USA)* 50:703–710, 1963.

CHAPTER 11

Is It Worth It?: A Personal Perspective

DEAN RAGONE

It was the evening of June 15, 1974. Just the day before I had completed my sophomore year in high school. I was looking forward to spending the summer with my family at the New Jersey shore, as I had done for 16 years. It had become a tradition in our area for my friends and I to get together to say our good-byes before everyone went their separate ways for the summer.

One of my friends was having a swimming party, and I was among the first to arrive. There I was, 16 years old, 5 feet 8 inches tall, and a healthy adolescent in every way. I was standing on the edge of the pool when someone suggested that we take a swim before the rest of the crowd arrived. On impulse, I dived headfirst into the pool—hitting the wall of the pool.

My head was under water. My arms dangled in front of my eyes. I couldn't feel any part of my body below my neck. I remember knowing that if I panicked I would drown, and I have always been taught never to panic, especially in water. I was under for at least a minute before my cousin Jeff noticed that I was in trouble and pulled me out. But, to this day, I can remember every second of that dreadful experience. I really did see my "life pass before me" from when I was a young child until that terrifying moment when so many visions raced through my mind as I held my breath. I even remembered how I had been so bored in history class the past semester that I had practiced holding my breath to build up my lung capacity for water skiing and surfing!

I was rushed to the local hospital where I laid in the emergency room on my back and unable to move at all. Shortly after I arrived, I became very sick to my stomach. I thought it was from the concussion that I kept reassuring my Mom that I had. She said I would be fine. The neurosurgeon ordered x-rays, and such great care was taken in transferring me to the x-ray table that I began to realize that this was much more than a concussion. It took four men to move me, including my two uncles and my father.

From the emergency department I was moved to the intensive care unit where I spent the next 15 days realizing that life was not a game, but an experience in which you continue to learn each and every moment. I had no feeling from my neck down. It was so frightening, lying there trying to understand what was happening to me.

Every morning the doctor would visit and question whether I could move my arms, my legs, and my hands and if I could feel the pins that he stuck into me. Every day the answer was "no" to everything he asked. After the eighth day, the neurosurgeon called in a physiatrist to evaluate my progress (which was nil) and to determine the type of rehabilitation center to which I should be referred. The physiatrist also offered his own opinion of my prognosis.

That day was very important to me and to my family. The doctor performed a very thorough examination from head to toe and then he told me that, as a result of my broken neck, I would remain paralyzed from my shoulders down for the remainder of my life. He said it was best that I be told in that manner so that I would just accept my injury and prepare for a new life-style.

Sixteen years old and more than a little confused about everything that had happened in the past week, I couldn't accept his tone or his words. After he left the room, I asked the nurse to get my mother. When she walked in I explained what the doctor had said and started to cry for the first time since the accident. She tried her best to console me, but the impact of the doctor's words was too much for me to overcome.

The doctor had recommended several rehabilitation centers, and my father and my uncles checked out each one. They all agreed that the best for me was the medical center with a large rehabilitation unit. And so, I was transferred there just 2 weeks after my injury.

The first few days at the rehabilitation center were a fiasco. Because of the paralysis, I had no control over my bowels or bladder. They had inserted a catheter into my bladder the first day I was injured and told me that I must "push" fluids to prevent infection. Unfortunately, I came down with a nasty infection during my first days of rehabilitation.

So there I was—a new patient in a whole new environment with a fever of 103°! This was to be the beginning of my rehabilitation and the beginning of a whole lot of new problems. I was fortunate to have a resident doctor who took pride in his job. He stayed with me for 24 hr until my fever subsided. I was getting antibiotics and was placed on an ice mattress (with which I became very acquainted during my stay).

I was very lucky to have my mother and my aunt stay with me that night, too. Although they were very scared at the time, they were able to put on a great act. In fact, throughout my rehabilitation program, my entire family put on a great act. They maintained a positive attitude throughout my many setbacks—at least in front of me.

After my fever dissipated, I was moved to a room with three other patients. My parents would have preferred a private room for me, but I liked the idea of having roommates.

During the first month, I developed repeated bladder infections and blood clots in my left leg that moved to my lung. All of that delayed the operation on my neck by 3 weeks. When it was finally done, the doctors considered it a great success. They fused my fifth and sixth cervical vertebrae with bone that they took from my hip. Soon after the operation, some feeling began to return throughout my body, and there was some improved movement of my left arm. Most peculiar of all, at that point I was able to move my toes! Needless to say, this brought much enthusiasm to my family and to me.

As a result of all of my complications and the postoperative recuperation, my first 2½ months were spent in bed. I also lost 30 pounds. I hadn't had much of an appetite through all of it. My family would see me during visiting hours, and one of my aunts who worked a few blocks away in the city would visit during her lunch hour. They all brought me all kinds of treats. One day my aunt arrived with a pizza, and from that day on, I had a great appetite—for pizza! I quickly gained back all of the weight I had lost, and then some. At the same time, I was beginning to feel more physically fit, although my overall improvement was still coming along very slowly.

Having never been in a hospital before, I was surprised to find such dedicated nurses who worked very hard at making me as comfortable as they could. The relationship I acquired with them helped me adjust to the environment around me. To this day, I believe that they were a main ingredient to making the rehabilitation process more comfortable for me. I can actually say that throughout all of the problems back then, there was also much laughter that will always remain part of my many fond memories of the nurses.

My day always began with the sound of the nurses waking me up and preparing me for the visit from my doctor. I felt very fortunate to have a doctor who not only had "class" and understanding but who also treated me as an adult. From the very beginning, when I began to see improvement he would show little emotion, but he always had a special sparkle in his steel-blue eyes. His famous response to my questions was always, "Time will tell." He never had a negative attitude, but at the same time he was very careful not to appear overly optimistic.

I always valued his opinion and still do to this day. He had very subtle ways of making suggestions without sounding negative. For instance, one day when I was able to move my arm enough to position a book I was reading, he asked me if I enjoyed reading. I responded, "Yes," and he proceeded to explain how important it was for me to use my brain. Because of my injury, my priorities would begin to change. Fortunately, I was only 16 years old and still young enough to alter my future plans without a major hardship. Unlike a man of his forties who had worked as a carpenter all his life, my adjustment to the injury should be less difficult.

And so I realized that I must prepare myself in case my return was limited, even though my goal was complete recovery. Education must be a priority in the event that I could only depend on the function of my brain. My parents had always encouraged education, the doctor wanted the best for me, and I realized they were right. I began my junior year of high school being tutored in the hospital.

After the doctor's morning visit, which consisted of the muscle test, the pin pricks and a general examination, it was time for physical therapy. The first day of therapy was very traumatic. I knew I was incapacitated and therapy was going to be a challenge—but after 2 months in bed, I was expecting an instant cure. I had some movement of my arms, but they were still very weak. I knew that if I could lift weights it would just be a matter of time before I became stronger. Well, was I in for a surprise!

My therapist was a very young, petite girl who was very sure of herself. I felt she was going to have her hands full with me. She transferred me to a mat to test my trunk balance. I tried to sit supporting myself with my arms and I kept falling over. With every try I got more discouraged, but by the end of the week, I was able to throw a knit ball underhanded while sitting long-legged. Wow! What a big accomplishment!

The therapist was so pleased that she invited my mother into the therapy room to see what I had accomplished. Years later, my mother told me that it was heartbreaking for her to watch her once healthy, athletic son begin a whole new way of life that day. She knew that it would be a hard struggle, and my family was ready to share it with me.

As the weeks passed there was more improvement. My goal at that time was to be able to wheel my own chair. I kept seeing other patients wheeling, and I set a goal to do the same. When I finally got a chair with lugs on the rims (because I couldn't grip the rims), I was ecstatic. I thought, "Look out, here I come!" To my dismay, like everything else, it was harder than it looked. I was only able to roll about 10 feet in a full minute. It took much time and endurance to wheel the chair from my room to therapy, but it gave me some independence, and that was psychologically important to me. Looking back now, I would say that was my first attempt to gain some semblance of independence.

Besides learning to sit and to wheel the chair, there were many phases of physical therapy that took total concentration and perseverance. Shifting my buttocks a few inches on the mat was an arduous task for me—although it may seem trivial to anyone who does it all the time without thinking.

Every few weeks my therapist tested my muscles to see how I was progressing. Even though it was 4 months since I had been injured, I was still confused by the injury. I was considered to be a "C5-C6 quad." However, I was "incomplete," and that is why I got some return below the level of the spinal cord that had been injured.

I was really confused by the spasticity that I was experiencing. There were times when I would be lying in bed, and all of a sudden, my legs would move. The first time it happened, I thought I was getting movement back. I immediately called the nurse, only to learn that this type of involuntary movement was a result of the injury.

The more intense therapy I received, the more spasticity I encountered. My legs would shake for hours. At times my legs were so stiff it required two people to break the spasms. Although I thought the spasms were a hindrance at first, in time I found that I could make them work for me. But initially the spasms could only be controlled with Valium. I disliked the Valium because it made me very tired and I was unable to complete my therapy sessions. I slept most of the time. The doctor suggested that I try Lioresal, a drug that was still experimental at that time—and it worked great. I was able to participate in therapy and still be awake when my family visited.

I was very intense during the therapy sessions, but at times, they seemed like a mountain that was too high to climb. It just took so much time to be able to do the most minute things, such as trying to feed myself and brushing a fly from my face. There were many times when I wondered if it was all worth it . . .

Because I had therapy 5 days a week, I had weekends to recuperate and enjoy my friends and family when they visited. They would give me support and encouragement to face the coming week.

After 3 months in the hospital, the doctors and nurses decided I was ready to go home for a weekend. The nurses explained to me and my family what was to be done for me while I was at home. It was a tremendous task. My family tried to prepare for the weekend that would be a test of how they would adjust to me.

As the ambulance drove up to my house I heard firecrackers and saw my family and friends waiting to greet my homecoming. I felt embarrassed and uncomfortable, and I couldn't wait to get inside the house. It was the first time since my injury that I didn't want anyone around me except my family. I knew everyone was happy for me to be home, but I became angry for the fuss everyone made. As always, my mother took most of the blame, but she always understood my feelings and moods.

All I could think about was that I wanted to be back in the hospital where I had become accustomed to the environment. As the evening progressed, I became more comfortable in my home. I had been gone for 3 months, and it seemed like nothing had changed.

The house was a split-level—not very good for someone in a wheelchair. My father's den and the patio on the first floor had been converted for me, and so I had all the conveniences I needed even though I couldn't return to "my" room.

Besides being just barely able to maneuver my chair and hardly able to feed myself, I was completely dependent on my family for round-the-clock care. During the night, my mother got up every 2 hr to turn me so that I wouldn't develop bed sores (which I never developed, fortunately).

In the morning she had to bathe and dress me with the help of her sisters who both lived just next door. They also had to take care of my catheter by flushing it out to make sure that it didn't clog. This was all new to them, but believe me, they handled everything like pros. I know that if they didn't understand something they at least knew just how to handle it so that they didn't frighten me. I was easily frightened then. I had come to trust the nurses who cared for me everyday and anyone else made me very hesitant.

And, my first weekend at home was a success, right? Wrong. The one thing about the injury is that there is no such thing as everything going as planned. On Sunday I awoke feeling fine, knowing that I would be back in the hospital by six o'clock. By early afternoon, though, I began to sweat. Soon I had soaked my shirt and within minutes I had a pounding headache. I never had had such a pain in my head.

My mother quickly called the hospital. The nurse told her that the catheter was probably clogged and that she should try to flush the catheter. Well, she tried, but it remained clogged. I was rushed back to the hospital by ambulance. As far as I was concerned they couldn't move me fast enough because the pain was unbearable.

When I arrived at the hospital, the nurse pulled my pants down, pulled out a pair of scissors, and cut the catheter. Urine poured out like a fountain. What a mess . . . but what a relief! Within minutes, my blood pressure was down and the headache was gone. The nurse explained that what had happened was that the catheter became clogged and the bladder had become overdistended. It's called "autonomic hyperreflexia." And so my first visit home resulted in a new problem, something else for me to be concerned about.

As the weeks went by, I began to get more function in my arms, but my hand dexterity wasn't improving. I think the poor dexterity in my hands was probably due, in part, to my attitude toward occupational therapy. From the very first day I entered occupational therapy, I had formed some sort of denial.

First of all, I wanted more physical therapy because I thought that would make me stronger. Occupational therapy just seemed to keep me from physical therapy.

The other reason for my poor attitude was that I was still 16 years old and somewhat immature. When I first saw what took place in occupational therapy it reminded me of my kindergarten days. They had all these ceramic fixtures I could paint, as well as pegs to place in the holes of a board. I kept telling myself how boring it was, especially for a quad like myself.

It took me a long time to realize that occupational therapy is vital in helping with independent living skills. Everything that went on in OT had a double meaning. The occupational therapist was able to help me by letting me paint with the brush held between my fingers. At the same time as I was improving the dexterity in my hands, I was enjoying the activity. Occupational therapy is an integral part of the rehabilitation process, but for me, it didn't take effect until after I left the hospital and could understand how it had helped.

Six months after the accident I was still improving in therapy. My health had stabilized to the point where the doctors, nurses, and therapists thought that it was time for me to leave the hospital and begin my new life at home. I was very confident even though I couldn't do very much. I felt secure in the hospital environment, which may sound crazy. The 24-hr care and all the attention I got in the hospital made me prefer to stay there, rather than go home.

But it was time to leave. My discharge was scheduled for the week before Christmas. The day they told me, I began to reflect on my stay there. I knew I had entered as a youthful 16-year-old who knew nothing about spinal cord injury. Now I was a 17-year-old who had grown up quite quickly and knew nearly every function of the body.

One thing that amazed me about my injury was how my bowel and bladder had been affected. At first I didn't have control over either. After 4 months of an indwelling catheter, I was told that it was time to train my bladder to function on its own again. The first step was to be catheterized every 4 hr. That meant that I would be without a catheter in me. However, I was introduced to an external catheter. When a nurse first described it to me I laughed and didn't believe such a thing existed. Was I in for a surprise!

From the first day I used an external catheter until I was finally able to go without it, I felt trapped. I despised it and it affected me to the point where I couldn't accept it even though I was grateful that my bladder function was returning. Sure, it was a convenience and there was no alternative, but to me, it was socially undesirable. There were many things about my injury that I could accept. For some reason, though, the external catheter hindered me mentally.

I was very fortunate that eventually I began to have control of my bladder. But in order to be bladder-trained, I had to wear the external catheter. I was in a "Catch 22" situation. I was aware of my bladder at all times. I learned to heed the signals my body presented, such as cold sweats, in order to eliminate the need for the external catheter. To help facilitate my voiding, I was taught to palpitate my bladder. Within 3 years of my injury, I was completely free of the external catheter. Since then, I have had complete control, and my motto has been, "Have bottle, will travel."

Compared to my bladder program, the bowel retraining program was easy. I started off with a Dulcolax tablet every morning—which is comparable to "Liquid Plumber" at times—and 8 hr later a suppository was inserted. I now only use a suppository when it is needed.

I had my unusual episodes in the hospital, both good and bad. Reflecting over my 6-month stay in the hospital, I knew that my whole outlook on life had changed. I had learned to be more patient and to have more perseverance and endurance. These things have remained with me over the years.

The day I left the hospital I was extremely depressed. I was frightened to leave the hospital environment. I had grown to love many of the nurses and aides who took so much of their personal time to help me through the most traumatic period of my life. And I knew then that the hope I had of walking out of the hospital had not materialized.

Although I made great strides since I was first injured, I was still dependent on others for assistance. The doctor had recommended that I continue therapy at home. My parents had contacted a local therapist who had a gym near my home. Now my life in the hospital was behind me, and it was time to enter the real world to see how I could perform.

The rehabilitative process is one that not only encompasses the traditional therapies but also includes very important support groups, such as family and friends. Having family support, my adaptation to the new environment made life somewhat easier than I initially expected. When I arrived home, I still had mixed emotions, but I knew there were other goals for me to reach. I felt very comfortable at home that first week because of all the attention that was being shown me. My physical therapy program wouldn't start until after Christmas.

I was in very good spirits as Christmas approached. My mother planned a big party for all my relatives and friends on Christmas Eve. Early in the evening I felt very strong and wanted to try to stand up on my own two legs. When I told my parents what I wanted to do they were surprised—speechless and apprehensive. They were afraid for me to try, because if I failed, it could result in a night of depression instead of the happy occasion that was planned. They asked me to wait for my uncles to arrive, and I said that was fine with me.

The apprehension of seeing so many people who had not seen me lately and the decision to try to stand increased the spasticity in my legs. I knew then that I would succeed. The spasms were strong, and with my faith and trust in God, I knew I could do it.

When my aunts and uncles arrived, they knew I was up to something because I was sitting there with a big smirk on my face. Without hesitating, I immediately told them of my plan. They were surprised and willing to help. They were as excited as I was. My father and uncle grabbed me under the arms, someone pulled up on the back of my pants, and the ladies pushed on my knees. Within seconds, they had me standing with my legs locked in a spasm that even Charles Atlas couldn't have broken!

I was up for about 30 seconds before I became dizzy. They sat me back in the chair and my legs shook for nearly 10 min. Now I knew that I had something to work with—and something to work for! I was so pleased that I repeated the performance later in the evening.

From that day on I stood until I couldn't tolerate it any more. My father had a carpenter design and build a standing box to fit my proportions exactly so that my knees wouldn't buckle.

After Christmas, I began working with Jim, my therapist. I was frightened at first, but Jim taught me very quickly that I had no time to be frightened. He had such great descriptive adjectives for me the first day that I knew he meant business. Within an hour he had called me every name in the book—including some I'd never heard. His least offensive adjective was "puke" (which became my "handle" at the gym—and now even my little godchild refers to me as the "puke").

Jim was a strong believer in weight-lifting. Unfortunately for me, my hand grip was not good enough to grasp the weights. However, he was able to get me to use my palms on the Universal gym equipment. This was the real world. Jim devoted an hour and a half of straight work to me. It was all business. The therapists in the hospital had been beautiful, caring people who did the best they could. But they had other patients to attend to, and I had had time to take it easy. Not so with Jim. When I got home that night all I wanted to do was sleep. When I awoke the next morning my arms were sore. Thank goodness, Jim believes in weight-lifting every *other* day.

When I arrived at the gym, I was lifted out of my wheelchair and sat up against the wall. Jim said he wanted to test my balance. He then proceeded to nudge my shoulders until I fell to my side. He repeated it until I was able to give him some resistance. I was elated. (The thing about this injury is that, if you don't try something, you don't know what ability you have.) After about 15 min, Jim gave me a long rest break.

After the break, Jim asked me how I felt and I told him, "Great." And so he asked me to move my arms in front of my face while I sat against the wall. It took some concentration, but I was able to do it.

The next day he had me continue this "shadow-boxing" exercise, as well as the weight-lifting. After a brief rest, he came back into the room with three basketballs.

I knew exactly what he had in mind. If there was ever a time for an instant cure, I was all for it. My legs immediatley went into spasm. All I could think of was what a broken nose must feel like. Jim proceeded to throw the basketballs at me, and I did my best to block them. Fortunately, my nose was not broken. I was really proud of myself. Jim was unorthodox in his methods, to say the least—but that was fine with me.

As the weeks progressed, so did I. Not only was I going to the gym every day, but I was being tutored at home and, most importantly, standing in my standing box every night. It was great to feel pressure on my feet. Within a month's time, I was able to stand for a half-hour at a time.

Standing for a half-hour was boring, but fortunately, I had a family that really sacrificed for me. Every single night, my father and uncles would put me in the box, and my mother and aunts would be there to keep me company. They would review my homework, watch television with me, and cheer me on. I amused myself by learning to do "push-ups" while standing in the box.

After 2 months at home, I was pretty much settled into my new environment and routine. I was happy with my improvement and doing well with my school work. I really wasn't accepting my injury, though. I was still insecure around my friends and never allowed any of them to help me with therapy.

I had some great friends, and even though I avoided them, they still hung in there with me. I did lose two childhood friends. I think they just couldn't deal with my injury, and I don't fault either of them. I met up with one of them years later in college, and we have renewed our friendship. It was almost 2 years before I felt comfortable around my friends, but as the years went by, I overcame it. Now I find myself to be very comfortable with my friends and even strangers.

Jim liked the idea of the standing box. He believed that my upper body had to get stronger. He wanted to get me up on parallel bars. I had advanced from basketballs to tennis balls. At home I was still dependent on my mother and father for my daily personal care and turning every 2 hr at night. The dexterity in my hands had improved to the point where I was able to write, feed myself, brush my teeth, and do other little things for myself. I still had to master dressing myself, and that would take a little more patience to accomplish.

One night late in February, I made another spontaneous decision. It was time to try to walk. I knew that I could move my feet a little while sitting in the chair, but to do it standing would be something altogether different.

I had my father and uncles hold me up. I was used to standing by then, and so it wasn't bad at first. Spasms took over when I tried to move my right leg. My legs moved like an astronaut's in space. I walked about 10 feet. We all laughed at how funny I looked—and with much happiness because I had walked at all. It was a joyous occasion for all of us. My mother would tell me later that all she could picture at that moment was my crossing the street in "space steps."

I knew that with the return of new muscles and the increased use of those muscles, my spasticity would play a crucial role in ambulation. The object was to control the spasms and not get rid of them completely. At the time I took those space steps, I realized that I had a lot more work to do to make my arms stronger too. I was working hard on the weight machine three times a week, but I couldn't get them stronger fast enough. I was still working without my triceps, but my biceps and deltoids were becoming stronger all the time. I felt mentally strong too.

I attribute much of my mental strength to Jim, my physical therapist. He made me tough mentally through some very unorthodox means. There were days when he would have me crawling through the locker room full of people. He wasn't doing it to embarrass me, but to force me to feel comfortable around people. His methods weren't from textbooks, but they worked for me.

Jim was elated to hear that I was able to take some steps. He and an assistant stood me up, and again I took some space steps. Jim became a little overconfident and decided to release his hold on me. Fortunately, his assistant was still holding on, or I would have been on the floor in a hurry. Of course, with every motion Jim has a reason. This time he wanted me to conquer my fear of falling. He was preparing me for the inevitable.

It was the latter part of March and I was progressing rapidly. My father had a set of parallel bars made for me, and they were set up in the family room at home. At first, I was hesitant to use them, not trusting my arms to support my body. But my legs were able to give me more support than I had thought. Using the parallel bars, I was able to take smaller, more controlled steps. I worked with the parallel bars for nearly 3 months.

Then I plateaued temporarily. I had strengthened all the muscles I had to work with at that point, and I just had to wait to see what (if any) other return I would get.

In the beginning of the summer I began to feel the heat. I noticed that my body could not withstand the heat as it used to. Jim decided that the best therapy at that time was swimming. I showed up for therapy on a hot day to attempt my first swim since I broke my neck the year before. As usual, Jim had his own idea as to how I should begin. He and my older brother lifted me from the wheelchair and threw me into the water.

I had no life preserver and no idea how to swim without the use of my legs and only partial movement in my arms. I tried to do the backstroke, using only my arms. From that moment on, I have never feared the water again. In fact, I now love to swim every opportunity I get.

As the summer progressed, I was feeling stronger than ever. I was still using the parallel bars at night and swimming and lifting weights during the day. Jim was anxious to see me try to walk with a walker now that my arms were stronger. I wasn't so sure.

Jim had me stand with him in the middle of a basketball court while he held the walker. I was so apprehensive that, no matter how much Jim told me to "move it," my spasticity increased and I became more frightened. As he lowered me to the floor it was one of the few times Jim gave in to me. But it didn't last. After a short rest, he had me up on my feet again, and he moved the walker as I moved my legs. It worked fine until the spasms in my legs prevented my keeping up with him. I was stretched out as far as possible and when I moved my left leg to follow my right I began to control the spasticity.

It took me about 2 weeks until I could finally move the walker myself. I was limited, but it was another new beginning. I practiced every night, learning to fall, as well as walk. Fortunately, I never had any serious injuries as a result.

My next goal was to get onto the walker without any assistance. I had to use what I call a "low bridge" walker and my own unorthodox style, but it works 99% of the time. A year and 3 months after I was injured I got to the point where I was able to walk from one room to another in my house. I had come a long way, but I still had a lot more to tackle.

I was building models to improve my hand dexterity. I had begun my senior year in high school being tutored at home. I was still socially inactive and depended on my mother and father for my everyday care. I was pleased with the progress I had made and anxious to see how much more return I would get.

My senior year in high school passed quickly. By June I was able to walk a 100 feet at a time. I wanted to receive my high school diploma *standing*. I had to attend graduation practice, and I was very apprehensive. I saw many friends I had not seen for 2 years.

The day of graduation was very special. It was 2 days before the second anniversay of my injury. My whole family and many friends were able to attend the graduation ceremony to help me celebrate this special event. It was very important to me that they were there, because they were responsible for *my* being there.

Although I had planned to stand to receive my diploma, earlier in the day I had chickened out. I was afraid that I would spasm out. When my name was called my two friends, Brian and Peter, pushed me up to the podium, and at the same time, the whole auditorium rose to give me a standing ovation. When I got back to where we had been sitting, I said to Brian, "I'm so embarrassed." His response was, "You loved it!" I thought for a second before I realized he was right.

The summer went by fast. I was working hard at the gym to increase my distance with the walker. My older brother Daniel was able to walk with me outside every evening.

I entered Rutgers University on September 8, 1976. I was very fortunate in that I lived only 6 miles from the school. Because my older brother was now in college away from home, I arranged for someone else to take me to school. For the first 2 years I attended only on a part-time basis.

I remember my first day of college as if it were yesterday. My first class was "Introduction to Psychology." I wheeled into the classroom and noticed that the only spot for me was across the room. However, there was a desk in my way. I tried to move the desk, but knocked it over instead. I couldn't pick it up, and so I left it and moved to my spot. Everyone in the room looked at me, and I felt very self-conscious, knowing all eyes were on me. The professor walked in looking like the stereotypical college professor—wrinkled jacket, tousled hair, and small wire-rimmed glasses.

The first day of college was my re-entrance into normal society. After 2 weeks I was very comfortable, and everyone was congenial with me. One day a student tried to be nice by opening an exit door for me. Unfortunately, the door led to a flight of stairs. I thanked him and explained that I thought the elevator might give me a smoother ride!

My next venture in college was to join an organization to fill the time between classes. I noticed an ad in the school paper for disc jockeys for the college radio station. I needed a push to the station because I wasn't sure where it was located, and when I finally reached the station, everyone was surprised and looked at me as if I were lost. I just smiled and said I wanted to be a DJ. The station manager seemed taken aback, but he explained that, if I could handle it, I would be on the air within a month's time.

Throughout my life, sports was a high priority for me. Nearly as important, I had always enjoyed music. The station manager seemed to be trying to appease me, and I knew that if I were to make an inroad into the studio it would depend on my ability to converse on the topic of music. Within a half-hour, I was in the studio checking out the control board. It had all sliding switches that would be easy for me to use. I practiced cuing up a record and did it like a pro.

My first day on the radio was another day of anticipation. I deliberated over what type of music to play. I had a long list of songs, but I needed a good lead-off song. I introduced myself on the air and played a classic that had a lot of meaning for me. It was "The Long And Winding Road" by the Beatles. Yes, it had been a long and winding road for me. I came a long way through trials and tribulations, but I still had a long way to go.

I played the music without any problems for an hour and a half. There were times, though, when I dropped records on the floor while the music was playing. During the 5 years on the radio, I never made a major faux-pas. I made many friends and enjoyed playing music from my own format.

My last day on the radio, I wanted to play a song that would summarize my experiences up to that time in my life. It was 1981, and oh, how my life had changed. The song I chose was "He Ain't Heavy, He's My Brother." The radio station had helped me associate and communicate with people. In the summer of 1980, my younger brother David and I had started a mobile disc jockey company called "C5-C6 Multi-Sound." We had had a lot of fun playing for private parties. The song seemed to say what I felt.

College life was good for me, although I didn't do very well academically the first year. I did finish my last four years with a 3.6 cumulative average and made the Dean's List several times. I was not a great student, and I had to study hard to make the grade. But reflecting over my 5 years of college, I know that I had come out of my shell.

By 1981 I was almost completely independent. I was still using the walker. With assistance, I was able to climb steps in the house to eat dinner with the family in the dining room. I continued to use the wheelchair whenever I left the house.

My next adventure was law school. My friend Tony had suggested that I attend with him. I applied and was scheduled to take the entrance exams. But I began to experience pain in my left leg. I was going to be admitted to the hospital for my yearly physical the day after the admission exams. The day of the exams, I awoke with excruciating pain in my leg and a high fever. My brother accompanied me to the examination, and I managed to pass the test! The next day they found a blood clot in my left leg, and I remained in the hospital for 6 weeks.

I began law school 3 weeks after I was discharged from the hospital. I regretted my law school decision after the first day. I struggled through two semesters. Some people may have been disappointed by my decision not to return for the second year, but I had proven to myself that I could do it. I just wasn't interested in law.

I had plateaued in my recovery at that point. I had grown to be a responsible person. I had begun many new projects and succeeded with them. Driving became a love for me. I traveled extensively throughout the United States. It gave me a strong feeling of independence and "normalcy."

The ability to drive gave me the opportunity for a larger social life. I became less dependent on others. Dating women became an easier task because I was able to escort them in my own automobile. Through my first 6 years I had been occupied with therapy, school, and adjusting and was not too inclined to date. But once the driving was conquered, I was less restricted, and my social life became very active. I also moved with my family into a new home that afforded me my own special living quarters.

When I began to date, it wasn't as difficult as I had feared. It was slightly awkward, but turned out well. After two dates, I realized that one young lady and I were not compatible. It was not only my insecurities, but a lack of interest on both our parts. Three months later, I was dating again.

At the New Year's Eve party, upon meeting my second girlfriend, we were both a bit shy. A few humorous remarks broke the ice, and by the end of the evening, I knew everything about her. As much as I liked her, I failed to get her telephone number. I managed to get it 2 weeks later, and after our first date, we became a steady couple.

We dated for 2½ years and it was great. She accepted my disability and was at ease with me. That relationship gave me confidence and helped me mature. Our breakup was a mutual decision. It was not due to my disability. We've remained friends to this day, and she has helped me in many ways that cannot be fully explained. I am very grateful that she entered my life when she did.

I had matured from a helpless 16-year-old boy to a mature college graduate. Apart from my family, my physical therapist Jim helped mold my character and mental attitude more than anyone else. It was because of him that I was able to feel good about myself. Without his support and that of my family, I believe I would be living in a nursing home like many other people I've seen since my injury.

My brothers have also been very attentive to my needs since my injury. My older brother Daniel is now a doctor of rehabilitation medicine. Despite all the problems that arose since my injury, the day he graduated from medical school was the happiest day of my life. My younger brother David was only 10 years old when I was injured. He has grown into a very responsible young man. My parents worked hard to make sure that he was not denied the attention due him, even though there were times when I needed more attention.

My friends too have become an integral part of my life. They have done so much for me by remaining loyal and faithful since my injury. I always tell people who have been injured that they should not shut out their friends, for they will understand and prove to be helpful in many ways.

It's funny, but I never told my friends about the external catheter, and I went through a lot of trouble to try to hide and disguise the legbag. One night, about 2½ years after the injury, I went out with some friends. We were drinking beer when my catheter came off, and I had a glaring accident! To minimize an embarrassing situation, I decided to use my disability to my advantage by deliberately spilling beer on my trousers. I think this quick thinking is part of a sixth sense that allows me to think faster and react accordingly to avoid the pain of embarrassement.

Throughout my incapacitation, I was fortunate to have only a few experiences of depression. I can attribute this to my environment and my trend of thought and attitude. I was pretty much optimistic about my recovery from the beginning. I always thought that whatever I did I had to give it my best. If something positive would come up, I would focus my concentration on that improvement.

My family has always been very spontaneous, and they never allowed me to be depressed. They made sure there was always some sort of activity going on, whether it was watching sports on television or going to a game. They sure kept me busy. Whenever I fell into a bit of depression, I just tried to think of someone who was worse off than I was and then set a new goal for myself. My mother always says, "Dean, you may have a handicap, but there are many young people out there without handicaps who are worse off than you!"

In the first stages of spinal cord injury, all sorts of thoughts go through your mind. It's very difficult to lie there and predict where you might be in 3 years. I didn't know what to expect from day to day. Although the first 2 years were like a dark cloud hanging over my head, that cloud wasn't permanent. Through rehabilitaton, the process of learning more about the injury helped the cloud dissipate. New priorities took over. I saw improvement as new goals were achieved. It was important to understand that all the initial problems would go away as long as I kept active and tried to keep an open mind.

Whenever I go out socially, I know that there are federal and state laws being enforced regarding accessibility. That makes me feel more comfortable. Even wheelchairs have become less institutional-looking. The new chairs are sporty-looking. lighter, faster, and take up less space, making me look less conspicuous. The first chair I had made me look like a tank.

The dark cloud that was once over my head is gone now. I have made tremendous strides. I am now a stockbroker. I am proud of my accomplishments.

Conclusions

When I was asked to write this chapter on whether rehabilitation is "worth it," I never gave it a second thought. I knew absolutely that it *was* worth it!!

There is one last point I would like to make. From the very first day of spinal cord injury, you are like a baby who must learn to do everything all over again. A whole new learning process begins. From the first day of therapy throughout the first 5 years, a molding takes place, gradual improvement occurs, but complete recovery may not happen.

Whatever return does appear, you learn to work with it. For example, I learned to use spasticity to my advantage. I worked to make my shoulder muscles and biceps stronger to compensate for the fact that my right triceps muscle doesn't work.

Rehab is a word used in the hospital, but it is a reality that must be applied the rest of my life. I don't exercise the way I used to, but I do try to keep myself in shape. Every time I show up at the gym I seem to run into someone who remembers what I looked like the first year I was there. They're always amazed at my improvement.

Rehabilitation is a continuing process. It's important to maintain some sort of exercise program to prevent the complications of inactivity. It's been a long and tedious road for me. Had it not been for the hard work and the love and support of my family and friends, I might still be lying in bed, being turned every 2 hr by my mother.

EDITORS' NOTE

There is no question that Dean's story is both typical and atypical. The daily rigor, emotional struggle, physical ups and downs, cyclical insecurities, and realistic and unrealistic hopes and dreams that he has described are common. The physical, mental, and spiritual effort required for anyone to maximize physical function successfully and adjust to physical limitations are well described in Dean's chapter. What makes Dean's story uncommon is the fact that financial resources and social supports have never been problems for him.

Far too many people who become spinal cord injured in our society are not so fortunate. Without adequate insurance coverage or sufficient personal wealth (which is extremeley rare), the overall rehabilitation program can be severely impaired. A vast number of persons with spinal cord injury do not have the financial resources to obtain even the basic equipment needed to assist them to achieve physical independence. Others may succeed in acquiring the basic equipment but are not able to provide for more than the most basic of needs, thereby achieving independence only within a limited environment. Rehabilitation is a costly process. Without the necessary financial backing, progress toward full independent living may be retarded.

Probably even more important than the issue of financial resources are the family and social resources that Dean described so vividly. With the constant, loving support of his family and friends, Dean has been able to survive the emotional ups and downs that are part of his life since his injury. Indeed, they have assisted him to become stronger because of them. This too is all too rare.

There is no question that family love cannot completely replace the need for adequate financial resources. But in many ways it can minimize the effects of limited resources on the overall outcome of disabling injury. With constancy in appropriate caring directed toward encouraging and fostering independence (as opposed to "doting"), family support can assist the person with spinal cord injury to reach beyond seemingly insurmountable financial limitations. Many instances could be recounted of people who seem to survive, thrive, and succeed, by virtue of their will alone. However, the value of support from family, friends, and society should not be underestimated in its ability to encourage the human spirit.

And so, although Dean's story is not necessarily typical, it is quite descriptive of the process and realities of life after spinal cord injury. Perhaps, short of cure, it is representative of the ideal outcome for comprehensive spinal cord injury rehabilitation and is indicative of the fact that the struggle *is* worth it.

Lorraine E. Buchanan, RN, MSN
Deborah A. Nawoczenski, M.Ed., PT

Index